T0226839

Revision Total Ankle Replacement

Editor

THOMAS S. ROUKIS

CLINICS IN PODIATRIC MEDICINE AND SURGERY

www.podiatric.theclinics.com

Consulting Editor
THOMAS ZGONIS

April 2013 • Volume 30 • Number 2

ELSEVIER

1600 John F. Kennedy Boulevard • Suite 1800 • Philadelphia, Pennsylvania 19103-2899

http://www.theclinics.com

CLINICS IN PODIATRIC MEDICINE AND SURGERY Volume 30, Number 2
April 2013 ISSN 0891-8422, ISBN-13: 978-1-4557-7143-1

Editor: Patrick Manley

Clinics in Podiatric Medicine and Surgery (ISSN 0891-8422) is published quarterly by Elsevier Inc., 360 Park Avenue South, New York, NY 10010-1710. Months of issue are January, April, July, and October. Business and Editorial Offices: 1600 John F. Kennedy Blvd., Ste. 1800, Philadelphia, PA 19103-2899. Customer Service Office: 3251 Riverport Lane, Maryland Heights, MO 63043. Periodicals postage paid at New York, NY and additional mailing offices. Subscription prices are $292.00 per year for US individuals, $410.00 per year for US institutions, $148.00 per year for US students and residents, $350.00 per year for Canadian individuals, $508.00 for Canadian institutions, $415.00 for international individuals, $508.00 per year for international institutions and $208.00 per year for Canadian and foreign students/residents. To receive student/resident rate, orders must be accompanied by name of affiliated institution, date of term, and the *signature* of program/residency coordinator on institution letterhead. Orders will be billed at individual rate until proof of status is received. Foreign air speed delivery is included in all *Clinics* subscription prices. All prices are subject to change without notice. POSTMASTER: Send address changes to *Clinics in Podiatric Medicine and Surgery*, Elsevier Health Sciences Division, Subscription Customer Service, 3251 Riverport Lane, Maryland Heights, MO 63043. **Customer Service: 1-800-654-2452 (US). From outside of the US, call 314-447-8871. Fax: 314-447-8029. E-mail: JournalsCustomerService-usa@elsevier.com (for print support); JournalsOnlineSupport-usa@elsevier.com (for online support).**

Reprints. For copies of 100 or more of articles in this publication, please contact the Commercial Reprints Department, Elsevier Inc., 360 Park Avenue South, New York, NY 10010-1710. Tel.: 212-633-3812; Fax: 212-462-1935; E-mail: reprints@elsevier.com.

Clinics in Podiatric Medicine and Surgery is covered in *MEDLINE/PubMed (Index Medicus)* and *EMBASE/Excerpta Medica*.

Printed and bound by CPI Group (UK) Ltd, Croydon, CR0 4YY
Transferred to Digital Printing, 2013

CLINICS IN PODIATRIC MEDICINE AND SURGERY

CONSULTING EDITOR
THOMAS ZGONIS, DPM, FACFAS

Contributors

CONSULTING EDITOR

THOMAS ZGONIS, DPM, FACFAS
Associate Professor, Fellowship Director in Reconstructive Foot and Ankle Surgery and Chief, Division of Podiatric Medicine and Surgery, Department of Orthopaedic Surgery, University of Texas Health Science Center San Antonio, San Antonio, Texas

EDITOR

THOMAS S. ROUKIS, DPM, PhD, FACFAS
Department of Orthopaedics, Podiatry, and Sports Medicine, Gundersen Lutheran Medical Center, La Crosse, WI, USA

AUTHORS

EVA ARLT, MD
Department of Orthopaedic Surgery, University Hospital Tübingen, Tübingen, Germany

JEAN-LUC BESSE, MD, PhD
Department of Orthopaedic and Traumatologic Surgery, Lyon-Sud Hospital, 69495 Pierre-Benite Cedex, France; Department of Orthopedic and Traumatologic Surgery, Université Lyon 1, IFSTTAR, LBMC UMRT-9406, Centre Hospitalier Lyon-Sud, 69495 Pierre-Bénite Cédex, France

FREDERICK F. BUECHEL Sr, MD
Professor of Surgery, Department of Orthopaedic Surgery, University of Medicine and Dentistry, Newark, New Jersey

JAMES K. DEORIO, MD
Associate Professor, Department of Orthopaedic Surgery, Duke University Medical Center, Durham, North Carolina

MICHAEL P. DONNENWERTH, DPM
Section of Podiatry, Department of Orthopaedics, Podiatric Medicine and Surgery Resident (PGY-III), Gundersen Lutheran Medical Foundation, La Crosse, Wisconsin

NORMAN ESPINOSA, MD
Department of Orthopaedic Surgery, Balgrist Hospital, University of Zurich, Zurich, Switzerland

MICHEL-HENRI FESSY, MD, PhD
Department of Orthopaedic and Traumatologic Surgery, Lyon-Sud Hospital, 69495 Pierre-Benite Cedex, France; Department of Orthopedic and Traumatologic Surgery, Université Lyon 1, IFSTTAR, LBMC UMRT-9406, Centre Hospitalier Lyon-Sud, 69495 Pierre-Bénite Cédex, France

MARK T.R. GADEN, MBBS, BMedSci, MRCS
Division of Orthopaedic and Accident Surgery, Nottingham University Hospital NHS Trust, Nottingham, United Kingdom

CARMEN I. LEICHTLE, MD
Department of Orthopaedic Surgery, University Hospital Tübingen, Tübingen, Germany

ULF G. LEICHTLE, MD
Department of Orthopaedic Surgery, University Hospital Tübingen, Tübingen, Germany

BRADLEY A. LEVITT, DPM
Instructor/Clinical and Fellow in Reconstructive Foot and Ankle Surgery, Division of Podiatric Medicine and Surgery, Department of Orthopaedic Surgery, University of Texas Health Science Center at San Antonio, San Antonio, Texas

CHRISTOPHE LIENHART, MD
Department of Orthopedic and Traumatologic Surgery, Université Lyon 1, IFSTTAR, LBMC UMRT-9406, Centre Hospitalier Lyon-Sud, 69495 Pierre-Bénite Cédex, France

GRAHAM MCCOLLUM, FCS Orth (SA), MD
The Institute for Foot and Ankle Reconstruction, Mercy Medical Center, Baltimore, Maryland

FALK MITTAG, MD
Department of Orthopaedic Surgery, University Hospital Tübingen, Tübingen, Germany

MARK S. MYERSON, MD
The Institute for Foot and Ankle Reconstruction, Mercy Medical Center, Baltimore, Maryland

BENJAMIN J. OLLIVERE, MBBS, BA (Oxon), MRCS (Trauma & Orthopaedics)
Division of Orthopaedic and Accident Surgery, Nottingham University Hospital NHS Trust, Nottingham, United Kingdom

MICHAEL J. PAPPAS, PhD
Professor Emeritus, Department of Mechanical Engineering, New Jersey Institute of Technology, Newark, New Jersey

MARK A. PRISSEL, DPM
Department of Medical Education, Podiatric Medicine and Surgery Resident (PGY-II), Gundersen Lutheran Medical Foundation, La Crosse, Wisconsin

THOMAS S. ROUKIS, DPM, PhD, FACFAS
Attending Staff, Department of Orthopaedics, Podiatry, and Sports Medicine, Gundersen Lutheran Healthcare System, La Crosse, Wisconsin

JOHN J. STAPLETON, DPM, FACFAS
Associate, Foot and Ankle Surgery, VSAS Orthopaedics, Chief of Podiatric Surgery, Lehigh Valley Hospital, Allentown; Clinical Assistant Professor of Surgery, Penn State College of Medicine, Hershey, Pennsylvania

ANDREAS SUCKEL, MD, Priv.-Doz.
Department of Orthopaedics and Trauma Surgery, Klinikum Stuttgart, Katharinenhospital, Stuttgart, Germany

CHRISTIAN WALTER, MD
Department of Orthopaedic Surgery, University Hospital Tübingen, Tübingen, Germany

STEPHAN HERMANN WIRTH, MD
Department of Orthopaedic Surgery, University of Zurich, Balgrist Hospital, Zurich, Switzerland

MARKUS WÜNSCHEL, MD, Priv.-Doz.
Department of Orthopaedic Surgery, University Hospital Tübingen, Tübingen, Germany

THOMAS ZGONIS, DPM, FACFAS
Associate Professor, Fellowship Director in Reconstructive Foot and Ankle Surgery and Chief, Division of Podiatric Medicine and Surgery, Department of Orthopaedic Surgery, University of Texas Health Science Center at San Antonio, San Antonio, Texas

Contents

Methodology for evaluation of total ankle replacements is described. Fusion and its problems are discussed as are those of total ankle joint replacement. Fusion is an imperfect solution because it reduces ankle functionality and has significant complications. Early fixed-bearing total ankles were long-term failures and abandoned. Currently available fixed-bearing ankles have proved inferior to fusion or are equivalent to earlier devices. Only mobile-bearing devices have been shown reasonably safe and effective. One such device, the STAR, has been approved by the Food and Drug Administration after a rigorous controlled clinical trial and is available for use in the United States.

Osteolysis is the loss of bone secondary to a pathologic process and remains the most common cause of failure of total ankle replacement. Friction at the bearing surface results in the generation of abraded wear debris of polyethylene. These activate a biologic cascade that may result in significant bone loss and subsequent loss of fixation of the prosthesis. Revision surgery must address this loss of bone and may be achieved through either bone grafting or use of appropriate revision prosthesis components.

We present a prospective series of 50 AES total ankle replacements performed between 2003 and 2006. The present report concerns medium-term results of cyst curettage-grafting. Twenty total ankle replacements underwent revision: 6 by tibiotalocalcaneal arthrodesis and 14 by cyst curettage-grafting. With 79% and 92% rates of unimproved or worsened functional and radiological status respectively, our results in cyst grafting are poor. No previous series of curettage-graft in evolutive periprosthetic total ankle replacement cyst have been reported. In periprosthetic cyst, we recommend annual radiological surveillance, with CT in case of cyst enlargement and/or increased pain, to allow implant removal and reconstruction-arthrodesis before collapse.

Total ankle replacement has become a popular treatment of symptomatic end-stage ankle osteoarthritis. Contemporary total ankle replacement systems provide more anatomic and biomechanically sound function. However, longevity is still limited and long-term results of modern total ankle replacement designs are not available. In the case of failure, conversion into arthrodesis has remained the treatment of choice but at the cost of hindfoot function and potential degeneration of the adjacent joints. Thus, revision total ankle replacement by exchange of the prosthetic components represents an attractive solution. This article focuses on revision total ankle replacement and conversion to ankle arthrodesis.

Although mid- to long-term results after total ankle replacement have improved because of available second- and third-generation devices, failure of total ankle replacement is still more common compared with total hip replacement and total knee replacement. The portfolio of available total ankle replacement revision component options is small. Furthermore, the bone stock of the tibiotalar region is scarce making it difficult and in some situations impossible to perform revision total ankle replacement. In these cases tibiotalar and tibiotalocalcaneal fusions are valuable options. This article describes which surgical procedures should be performed depending on the initial situation and gives detailed advice on surgical technique, postoperative care, and clinical results.

Failed total ankle replacement is a complex problem that should only be treated by experienced foot and ankle surgeons. Significant bone loss can preclude revision total ankle replacement and obligate revision though a complex tibio-talo-calcaneal arthrodesis. A systematic review of the world literature reveals a nonunion rate of 24.2%. A weighted mean of modified American Orthopaedic Foot and Ankle Society Ankle and Hindfoot Scale demonstrated fair patient outcomes of 58.1 points on an 86-point scale (67.6 points on a 100-point scale). Complications were observed in 38 of 62 (62.3%) patients reviewed, with the most common complication being nonunion.

The Agility total ankle replacement system was the most commonly performed implant in the United States for more than 20 years and has undergone four generations and seven phases of improvement. Much attention has been placed on intraoperative complications, such as malleolar fracture; nerve or tendon injury; and incision healing–related problems, such as wound coverage and infection. However, it is the intermediate- and

peripheral neuropathy and/or vascular disease are equally important and may alter the surgical approach to traumatic tarsometatarsal injuries. The initial diagnosis in the diabetic population may be delayed due to subtle radiographic findings and/or patient unawareness of trauma in the insensate foot. Failure to initiate treatment in the early stages of acute diabetic neuropathic Lisfranc injuries can predispose the patient to midfoot instability, potential ulceration, infection, and Charcot neuroarthropathy.

CLINICS IN PODIATRIC
MEDICINE AND SURGERY

Foreword
Revision Total Ankle Replacement

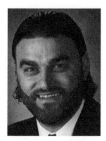

Thomas Zgonis, DPM, FACFAS
Consulting Editor

This edition of *Clinics in Podiatric Medicine and Surgery* is focused on revision total ankle replacement collaborated on by some of the most experienced surgeons around the world and under the scientific work of our guest editor, Dr Roukis. This edition completes the topic of total ankle replacement for addressing primary degenerative and posttraumatic ankle deformities as well as dealing with complications associated with various total ankle implants.

Various topics from management of aseptic and septic periprosthetic-related complications to subsequent ankle and tibiotalocalcaneal arthrodesis are covered in great detail with pertinent insights from our expert invited authors. Equal emphasis on surgical techniques and pearls in revision total ankle replacement from reimplantation to arthrodesis is accomplished for total ankle implants that are available in the United States.

Finally, I hope that this edition by our distinguished panel is helpful when dealing with complications arising from total ankle replacement. I would also like to thank the guest editor, invited authors, and publisher for making this project a reality and available to each reader.

Thomas Zgonis, DPM, FACFAS
Division of Podiatric Medicine and Surgery
Department of Orthopaedic Surgery
University of Texas Health Science Center San Antonio
7703 Floyd Curl Drive–MSC 7776
San Antonio, TX 78229, USA

E-mail address:
zgonis@uthscsa.edu

Clin Podiatr Med Surg 30 (2013) xv
http://dx.doi.org/10.1016/j.cpm.2013.01.004
0891-8422/13/$ – see front matter © 2013 Published by Elsevier Inc.

Preface

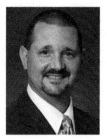

Thomas S. Roukis, DPM, PhD, FACFAS
Editor

It is with great pleasure that I serve as guest editor for this issue of *Clinics in Podiatric Medicine and Surgery* devoted to "Revision Total Ankle Replacement," which is the follow-up issue to "Primary Total Ankle Replacement" published in January 2013. My first consistent experience with total ankle replacement actually involved revision of failed Agility total ankle replacement systems (DePuy Orthopaedics, Warsaw, IN). As is now well known, this system is very demanding for primary implantation and the tolerance for malalignment or technical error is very small. The complications are many and, although some are relatively straightforward to manage, some are truly catastrophic with limited revision possibilities. It has taken me the past 5 years to truly understand the Agility and Agility LP total ankle replacement systems and the challenges associated with its revision enough to perform these complex surgeries well with regularity. Obviously, the Agility prosthesis is not the only total ankle replacement system that fails and requires revision. Simply put, it is the only one that has been implanted enough times and for a long enough period of time in the United States to demonstrate consistent failure of approximately 10%.[1] It should be noted that, throughout this *Clinics of Podiatric Medicine and Surgery* issue, revision will be defined as failure of the total ankle replacement system components sufficient to warrant manipulation and/or removal of the tibial and/or talar components with reimplantation using an alternative system or custom-designed implants; conversion to an arthrodesis; or amputation of the limb.

The intent of this issue is to provide up-to-date information available for the challenging problems associated with revision total ankle replacement. Little meaningful data are available in the world literature to guide treatment and I have gone directly to those who have published on this topic and asked them to provide us with meaningful approaches to revision total ankle replacement surgery. As one can see from the author list, this issue consists of an international "who's who" of revision total ankle replacement. These authors are to be commended for not only being on time with their submission but also for the wealth of detailed information they have freely delivered to you, the reader.

The modes of failure of current total ankle replacement systems are discussed first, followed by articles discussing approaches to aseptic and septic osteolysis

Clin Podiatr Med Surg 30 (2013) xvii–xviii
http://dx.doi.org/10.1016/j.cpm.2013.01.003
0891-8422/13/$ – see front matter © 2013 Published by Elsevier Inc.

podiatric.theclinics.com

management. Isolated ankle arthrodesis and tibio-talo-calcaneal arthrodesis following failed total ankle replacement are then discussed in detail, including a systematic review of the world literature. We then embark on management of the failed Agility, INBONE, and STAR total ankle replacement systems, again including a systematic review of the world literature specifically for the failed STAR prosthesis.

It is hoped that the readers of this issue of *Clinics of Podiatric Medicine and Surgery* will enjoy these articles and benefit from the surgical experience of the authors selected as much as I have.

Thomas S. Roukis, DPM, PhD, FACFAS
Department of Orthopaedics, Podiatry, and Sports Medicine
Gundersen Lutheran Medical Center
La Crosse, WI, USA

E-mail address:
tsroukis@gundluth.org

REFERENCE

1. Roukis TS. Incidence of revision after primary implantation of the Agility Total Ankle Replacement System: a systematic review. J Foot Ankle Surg 2012;51:198–204.

Failure Modes of Current Total Ankle Replacement Systems

Michael J. Pappas, PhD[a],*, Frederick F. Buechel Sr, MD[b]

KEYWORDS

- Ankle replacement • Ankle fusion • Fixed-bearing ankle • Mobile-bearing ankle
- Total ankle evaluation

KEY POINTS

- Food and Drug Administration (FDA) clearance of an ankle device does not imply safety because the FDA classification of class II for ankles is flawed.
- All of the FDA-cleared fixed-bearing ankle devices can, therefore, not be considered acceptable.
- All such devices available in the United States fail to satisfy reasonable design criteria because they all have serious design defects.
- None has acceptable, published clinical performance. Thus, these designs should not be considered for clinical use.
- Only the STAR, which has reasonable midterm and long-term results and FDA approval, seems preferable to fusion and acceptable for ankle reconstruction.

INTRODUCTION

Although there is much recent interest in ankle replacement for the treatment of severe ankle pathology, ankle fusion remains the current gold standard for such treatment. Still, a well-functioning, reliable, and durable replacement is preferable to fusion due to improved function, if for no other reason.

Unfortunately, most replacement ankle devices have been unsatisfactory[1–6]; thus, fusion remains the procedure of choice for most surgeons. There are, however, problems with fusion[7–9]; thus, there has been considerable effort in attempting to develop and market a satisfactory ankle replacement. Currently there are 4 ankle replacement devices generally available and in use in the United States. Three of these are 2-part devices, a tibial component with a bearing fixed to it and a talar component. These are the Salto Talaris by Tornier, the Inbone by Wright Medical Technology, and the Agility by DePuy. These devices are cleared by the FDA under a grandfather rule (510[k]) as substantially equivalent to devices available before July 1976. They are shown in **Fig. 1**.

[a] Department of Mechanical Engineering, New Jersey Institute of Technology, University Heights, Newark, NJ 07102-1982, USA; [b] Department of Orthopaedic Surgery, University of Medicine and Dentistry, 61 First street, South Orange Avenue, Newark, NJ 07079, USA
* Corresponding author. 8605 South Ocean Drive, Apartment 1203, Jensen Beach, FL 34957.
E-mail address: mjpappas32@comcast.net

Clin Podiatr Med Surg 30 (2013) 123–143
http://dx.doi.org/10.1016/j.cpm.2012.10.002
0891-8422/13/$ – see front matter © 2013 Elsevier Inc. All rights reserved.

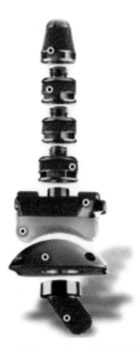

Fig. 1. Inbone Ankle. (Photo provided *courtesy of* Wright Medical Technology, Inc.)

One 3-part device, where the bearing is mobile with respect to the tibial and talar components, is available. This is the Scandinavian Total Ankle Replacement (STAR) ankle replacement (**Fig. 2**) by Small Bone Innovations, which has been approved by the FDA.

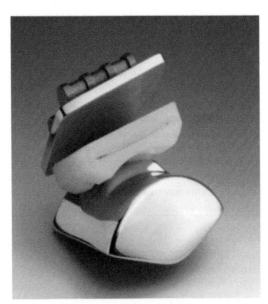

Fig. 2. The STAR ankle replacement. (*Courtesy of* Small Bone Innovations, Inc, Morrisville [PA]; with permission.)

The question is, Which of these devices, if any, is best suited to a patient's pathology and is preferable to fusion? This article provides a procedure for evaluating these implants and attempts to answer this question.

The devices on which the FDA determined, in 1982, the classification of allowable devices[10] were all failures and were withdrawn from the market.[11] The currently available 2-part devices cleared by the FDA were found "substantially equivalent" to those failed devices. Thus, the standard of proof required to show the acceptability of 2-part devices needs to be rigorous.

Three-part devices have, however, been significantly more successful and one such device, the STAR ankle, has completed a rigorous FDA controlled clinical trial and as a result been approved for general use.[12] Unfortunately, this clinical trial is short term. Fortunately, medium-term and long-term data suggest that this and other 3-part devices from European trials have shown promising results.[13–17]

This article evaluates the characteristics of these 4 devices to determine their suitability as effective ankle replacements. Furthermore, it compares them with fusion and other devices used in Europe.

EVALUATION METHODOLOGY

The evaluation of an orthopedic implant requires knowledge of the motion and stability of the joint involved, the forces on the joint, and the modes of failure possible for the device. In addition the evaluator needs to know the device characteristics and its clinical performance.

Motion of the Ankle

Ankle movement is a complex 3-D motion,[18] with infinity of instant axes of tibiotalar rotation, as is the case in all condylar joints. Fortunately, for purposes of analysis and design, the complex motion degrees can be approximated by a planar-plantar dorsiflexion,[19] axial (internal-external) rotation, and inversion-eversion.[19]

The 5° of freedom associated with the tibiotalar joint are illustrated in **Fig. 3**.

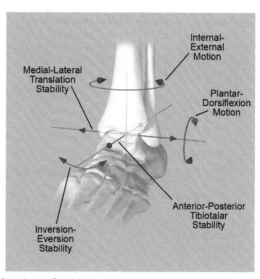

Fig. 3. Degrees of freedom of ankle motion and modes of ankle stability.

Plantar dorsiflexion

The normal plantar dorsiflexion range in level walking is typically approximately 25° to 35°. If limited, it adversely affects ankle function and can produce undesirable loading on the prosthesis, ligaments, and bone fixation interfaces.

Axial rotation

Normal axial rotation is approximately +5° to −3° during walking. Other activities can produce a maximum rotation of approximately 16°.[20–22] Any restriction of this motion is also undesirable because it produces undesirable torque on the prosthesis and bone fixation interface.

Stability

The tibiotalar joint is stable and, thus, is constrained against significant anterior-posterior, medial-lateral, and inversion-eversion motion. There are 2 types of stability: intrinsic stability, provided by the shape of the articulating surfaces, and extrinsic stability, provided by soft tissues.

Inversion-eversion

Normal inversion-eversion is approximately +10° to −2° during walking, although most of this motion is in the subtalar joint.[20–22] Inversion-eversion stability is provided by the tibiotalar ligaments and the width of the tibiotalar articulating surface (shown in **Fig. 4**).

Anterior-posterior

Anterior-posterior stability is primarily extrinsic and is provided by the ankle ligaments. Some intrinsic stability is also present.

Medial-lateral

Medial-lateral stability is almost entirely intrinsic and is provided by the ankle mortise. There is, however, approximately 2 mm of medial-lateral motion in the normal ankle.[20,21]

Forces

Tibiotalar compressive forces have been estimated to exceed 4 times body weight during normal walking. The posterior shearing forces are approximately 80% of body weight.[20]

The joint compression force is carried primarily by the tibiotalar articulating surfaces and partially by the talofibular joint. The anterior-posterior shearing force is carried by

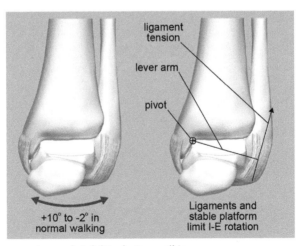

Fig. 4. Inversion-eversion and stability during walking.

these surfaces and the ligaments. The medial-lateral shearing forces are carried by the malleolar articulation and Inversion-Eversion torques by the articulating surfaces and ligaments.

The combination of the axial compression and shearing forces produce a peak resultant force vector on the tibiotalar joint, which is posteriorly inclined relative to the tibial axis as is the tibial articulation surface (shown in **Fig. 5**).

Failure Modes

The safety and reliability of orthopedic implant systems is of critical importance. Thus, it is essential to understand the modes and processes of failure and degradation of the elements of such systems and to determine the cause of failure when it occurs.

A thorough understanding of mechanical failure involves an understanding of the field of stress analysis,[23] corrosion, and wear.[24] A thorough understanding of stress analysis involves an understanding of material properties and the theory of elasticity.[25] Modern techniques for predicting the behavior of materials under loading allow reasonable prediction of such behavior if used in light of knowledge of material properties and elasticity theory.

An understanding of the risks of biologic failure is also essential. Such failure may occur in the absence of any damage to the implants by the release of toxic material from an implant by leaching or corrosion.[26] Biologic failure, however, is often associated with mechanical problems, such as loosening due to bone necrosis resulting from wear, or mechanical subluxation due to component subsidence.

Finally, complications can result from the surgical intervention. It is important, therefore, to understand such complications and methods for avoiding them.

Stress analysis

Stress analysis involves the prediction of stress and strain in a body under loading or thermal effects. Only the effects of loading are discussed.

Finite element analysis (FEA) was first introduced in 1943 by Courant using the Ritz numerical method and variational calculus to develop approximate solutions to a class of vibration problems, which, in 1956, Turner and colleagues expanded to include the deflection of complex structures.[27] Work over the past half century has expanded the

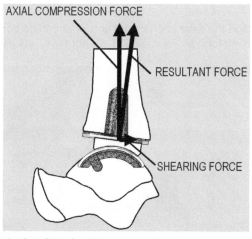

Fig. 5. Vector forces in the tibiotalar joint.

application of FEA and simplified its use. Linear FEA stress analysis of mechanical parts is now an integral part of most high-end computer-aided design (CAD) software packages. FEA may be used to analyze a mechanical part by creating a digital 3-D solid computer model of the part and then defining a mesh used to approximate the behavior of the part under the expected loading conditions.

To perform the analysis, an appropriate mesh is first generated with regions of expected high stress and stress concentration using a greater node density. Rigid body or elastic constraints are placed on the motion of those nodes where the part is attached to simulate its attachment boundary conditions and forces are placed on appropriate nodes to simulate the expected loading. A set of simultaneous differential equations is then formulated and solved computing the approximate stress and, if desired, strain or deformation at each node. The results are then presented, usually in graphic form to allow easy location of the largest stress and their values. This methodology is in common use by orthopedic implant designers.

Mechanical testing

The approximations used in analysis during design verification often make mechanical and clinical testing a requirement of validation studies. Mechanical test methodology is well defined by several American Society for Testing and Materials testing protocols developed by industry and the Society. It is usual to use these methods during the mechanical testing phases of verification and validation. Often, mechanical testing using these methods is required by regulatory authorities before approval of a device for general orthopedic use.

As a result of the sophisticated FEA stress analysis methods used and the development and use of standardized testing procedures, a high degree of reliability against fracture of the nonplastic components can usually be assumed.

Wear

The most serious mechanical complication is wear rather than fracture or deformation of the metallic elements of a device. An example of serious wear may be seen in **Fig. 6**, which shows the effects of various wear modes.

Polyethylene wear has received much attention due to catastrophic problems with metal-backed patellar[28,29] and tibial prostheses.[30,31] Such wear has been recognized by scientific investigators and clinicians as a major problem for some time.[32-37] Wear-related problems involve wear-through, breakup, and the physiologic effects of wear debris.[38,39]

To better understand the wear phenomena and what can be done to reduce wear and its undesirable effects an examination of abrasive, adhesive, 3-body, and

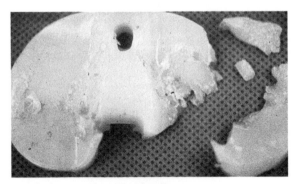

Fig. 6. Wear failure of a knee replacement bearing.

fatigue-related wear; contact pressures and stresses; and the relationship between design and wear is needed.

Abrasive Wear Abrasive wear results from direct contact between the metal and plastic components. Even polished surfaces are microscopically rough. If the metal is allowed direct contact with the plastic peaks (asperities) on the metal surface, it slowly gouges (abrades) away the plastic as the metal surface moves over the plastic surface, much as fine sandpaper abrades away a wooden surface. The rate of abrasion is a function of the smoothness of the metal surface; the rate declines as the height of the asperities declines (the metal becomes smoother).[40]

Human joint motion is characterized by a predominance of boundary and the more destructive dry lubrication. Boundary lubrication is improved, and the period of dry lubrication is reduced, if the wetting ability of the surfaces is increased.

Adhesive wear Adhesive wear results from localized welding and tearing, rather than gouging, of the contacting surfaces. When opposing asperities contact each other, the greatly localized nature of the contact produces such high stresses that the 2 materials in contact become welded or adherent. Translation of 1 with respect to the other then produces tearing or rupture of 1 or both of the asperities.

The wear rate under adhesive conditions is much higher than that associated with smooth surface abrasive wear. Such wear can apparently be minimized with ceramic against ultrahigh molecular-weight polyethylene (UHMWPE) articulations.[41]

Three-body wear The presence of contaminants, such as cement, bone debris, and loose metallic beads, as well as the wear debris of the articulating couple, also contribute to wear. This contribution is called 3-body wear.

Typically, the harder bodies become embedded in the soft bearing. These bodies then can rapidly abrade the metal surface increasing abrasive and adhesive wear. The much harder ceramic surfaces are more resistant to the effects of such contaminants.

Surface fatigue The dominant wear (perhaps better called fatigue failure) mode in knee replacements is fatigue related due to breakup under excessive fluctuating stress. Incongruent bodies in contact under load deform and produce an area of contact or a contact patch. The highest damaging stress, or von Mises stress, is approximately 1 mm below the surface of the UHMWPE near the center of the patch (**Fig. 7**).

As the metal component slides and rolls over the surface of the weaker plastic surface, the point of peak stress moves under the surfaces of the plastic. If the stress is high enough, cracks initiate below the surface. The cracks may then coalesce to produce pitting, delamination, and, by propagation through the part, catastrophic failure (**Fig. 8**). This is a classic mode of surface failure in rolling contact.[42] Such catastrophic wear is seen in **Fig. 6**.

Contact stress Ordinary FEA boundary conditions cannot be used to compute incongruent contact stresses because the deformation patch is not known and thus the analyst does not know where to apply node forces or what these forces are. Specialized software is needed to handle incongruent contact. Such software, although generally available, is expensive and not part of generalized mechanical CAD packages.

Fortunately, equations sufficient for use in incongruent knee prostheses, for the computation of the contact stress of 2 bodies in contact, were developed in the 1930s using elasticity methods.[42] Computations can readily be performed by a computational program, such as Mathcad. Considering the typically excessive

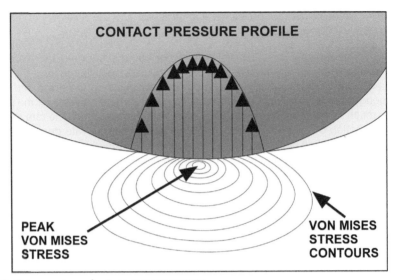

Fig. 7. Stress contours for incongruent contact.

stresses found in most ankle and knee designs, most designers are either unaware of such equations or disregard their teaching.

A theoretical and experimental study of contact stress[43] augmented with analysis of a mobile-bearing ankle and 2 fixed-bearing ankle devices demonstrates the superiority of the mobile-bearing tibiofemoral and tibiotalar articulations. Using a load of 2200 N, the contact stress is computed with the equations given in Seely and Smith[42] and used by Pappas and colleagues,[43] yielding the results shown in **Fig. 9**.

It may be seen that only the contact stresses in the area (mobile-bearing) type are within the recommended limit of 10 MPa.[44] The other (fixed-bearing) types have stresses greatly exceeding acceptable limits, even approaching or exceeding the compressive yield stress of UHMWPE, which is approximately 30 MPa.[45] In the wear testing of Pappas and colleagues,[45] it was found that the average wear of the fixed-bearing knees tested was 6 times greater than the mobile-bearing LCS (DePuy Inc, Warsaw, IN) knee tested.

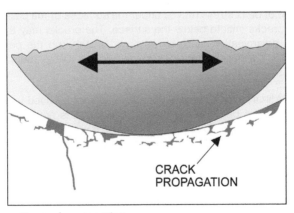

Fig. 8. Crack formation and propagation.

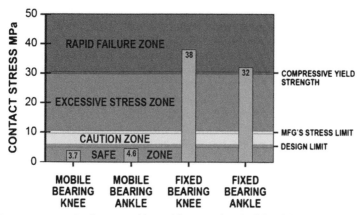

Fig. 9. Contact stresses in the B-P ankle and knee and typical fixed-bearing devices.

Misconceptions

Several misconceptions are prevalent on the effects of congruency and incongruency:

1. Incongruent surfaces become more congruent with use.
2. Mobile bearings have greater wear because they have wear on 2 articulating surface couples.
3. If a bearing is at least 6 mm thick, it is acceptable.
4. Mobile-bearing ankles are less stable.
5. Extrusion of the bearing is a significant complication.

These concepts are all unrealistic and untrue, as shown by Buechel and Pappas.[46] With respect to items 4 and 5, at least with respect to the B-P Ankle (Endotec, Inc, Orlando, FL), this device is more stable than most fixed-bearing devices and bearing extrusion is rare and was always the secondary result of talar component subsidence.

Other wear-related design considerations

Provision for adequate axial rotation It is a simple matter to produce a fully congruent design. Congruency, by itself, however, is not sufficient. This is evidenced by some of the early designs, which fail to provide adequate provision for axial rotation.[47] Mobility is needed along with congruity.

Provision for abduction Inversion of the ankle occurs during the swing phase of the walking cycle and during other normal activities. Although loads during the swing phase are low, they are still significant. To minimize wear, the articulating surfaces must accommodate such motion.

Biologic Failure

Just as mechanical failure leads to poor function, biologic failure of an artificial joint replacement can lead to significantly worse complications or even death. The most commonly encountered biologic failure modes are infection, osteolysis, progressive osteoporosis, avascular necrosis, periprosthetic fracture, and tumor formation.

Infection

Septic joint replacements occur in 1% to 2% of cases overall.[48] The gram-positive organisms of Staphylococcus aureus and S epidermides are most common and generally believed to occur at the time of initial surgery or shortly afterward if the skin incision fails to heal in a timely fashion.

Osteolysis

Small (submicron) polyethylene or metallic wear particles incite an inflammatory process, whereby macrophages and giant cells phagocytose the particles and attempt to digest them with lyzozymes and proteolytic enzymes. Unfortunately, the wear particles persist in the cytoplasm of these cells and continue to stimulate diges-tive enzyme production, which spills over into the surrounding bone and begins to digest this host bone. Once enough bone is lost in this osteolytic process, a cystic cavity filled with these macrophages and giant cells replaces the normal bone and begins to expand if the threshold for particle volume is exceeded.

If the osteolytic cysts become too large, then fixation failure of the implant can occur, requiring revision, curettage, and bone grafting of these defects to regain stability and function.

Progressive osteoporosis

Disuse atrophy of the bone, also known as progressive osteoporosis, occurs when a patient fails to load the bone sufficiently to maintain its strength and integrity. Regardless of the reason, such as a stroke, the host bone atrophies around the joint replacement and the device may loosen or the surrounding bone may fracture due to its weakened condition.

Avascular necrosis

Vascular compromise to supporting bone causes bone cell death, known as avascular necrosis or osteonecrosis. If the region of bone is in the talus, an ankle replacement fails due to collapse of the talar component into avascular bone.[49]

Such necrosis can be reduced by minimizing the interruption of the blood supply in the talus, as is commonly done by the resection of the talus in fitting the talar component.

Periprosthetic fracture

Although there is a mechanical component to fractures surrounding joint replacement implants, it is a failure of the bone that creates instability and can even be life threat-ening if sufficient fat emboli compromise cardiovascular function.

Tumor formation

Pseudotumors or malignant tumors can compromise a well-functioning joint arthro-plasty. Pseudotumors generally form from wear debris particles that accumulate.[50] Malignant tumors are rarely associated with joint replacement but have been reported to erode the bony fixation of implants, making them essentially unreconstructable.

Fixation

Component subsidence, particularly of the talar component, is a major complication of ankle replacement. Thus, a properly designed device should require minimum bone removal because the bone with the greatest load-bearing capacity is adjacent to the articulating surfaces and minimal resection results in minimal disruption of the blood supply to the load-bearing regions.

Clinical Results

The considerations (listed previously) are useful in evaluating ankle replacement devices but the best evidence of device longevity and function is their clinical perfor-mance. Buechel and colleagues formulate the simple, necessary, but not sufficient, conditions for orthopedic implant acceptability.[51] These are

1. There is reliable clinical evidence of 90% survivorship at 10 years.

2. The peak articulating surface contact stresses must be below 10 MPa during walking.

In addition, the surgical procedure and instruments used need to be analyzed to attempt to reduce the incidence of surgically introduced complications.

FUSION

Due to the historically generally poor performance of total ankle replacement (TAR), arthrodesis remains the procedure of choice for most orthopedic surgeons for ankle reconstruction. There seems, however, to be little literature on the long-term outcome of such a procedure. The data of Coester and colleagues[9] are unreliable, except to show a major loss of functionality in the fused joint due to the high loss to follow-up rate of 64% (41 of 64). Buchner and Sabo[52] in their average 9-year study of 48 patients found substantial pain relief, but a significant number (21%) of patients still had severe to moderate pain after fusion. Furthermore, their study found a failure rate defined as the need for reoperation of 19%.

These clinical studies demonstrate that ankle fusion is much less successful than total hip or knee replacement, where a 90% success rate can reasonably be expected with appropriate designs.

FIRST-GENERATION FIXED-BEARING TOTAL ANKLES
Clinical Outcomes

On July 2, 1982, the *Federal Register* published the Rules for Ankle joint metal/polymer semiconstrained prosthesis.[10] The Orthopedic and Rehabilitation Devices Panel of the Medical Devices Advisory Committee found that there was sufficient scientific evidence to support a class II designation. The Panel based its recommendation on 4 oral presentations based on 4 semiconstrained ankles presented by their developers.

The FDA agreed with the panel's recommendations and sought additional data and information on the safety and effectiveness of these devices. The FDA cited the following studies on 3 additional devices: those of Stauffer,[53] Scholz,[54] and Waugh and colleagues.[55]

The decisions of the panel and the FDA to designate semiconstrained ankles as class II were founded on these short-term encouraging results of early ankle designs based on presentations and publications of the developers of these ankles. Such a designation, particularly in light of what is known today, is unreasonable because these references and presentations cannot be considered reasonable proof of device safety and efficacy.

Longer-term studies, furthermore, demonstrate that these ankle types were failures. The performance of such ankles is illustrated in **Table 1**.

Analysis

Early ankle failures were primarily the result of excessive constraint, abetted by excessive contact stresses, and excessive bone removal, resulting in component loosening and subsidence.

Neufeld and Lee[59] state, "After early successes, the longer-term results bred failure." Lachiewicz and colleagues[60] reported on 15 patients with one of the most widely used prostheses, the Mayo ankle, with an average follow-up of 3.3 years and excellent results. When Unger and coworkers[56] reported on the same 15 patients with a longer follow-up of 6.2 years, deterioration in their clinical scores and radiographs was apparent.

Table 1
Long-term results of typical early fixed-bearing ankle replacement

Authors	Device	Number of Cases	Diagnosis	Average Follow-up	Survival Rate (%)
Jensen and Kroner,[1] 1992	TPR	148	SA (21), OA (2), RA (125)	4.9 y	48
Kitaoka et al,[3] 1994	Mayo	79	SA (65), OA (14)	5 y, 10 y, 15 y	79, 65, 61
Kitaoka and Patzer,[2] 1996	Mayo	168	RA (96), SA (64), OA (8)	9 y	64
Wynn and colleagues,[4] 1992	Beck-Steffee	30	RA (18), SA (12)	2 y, 5 y, 10 y	73, 40, 10
Helm and Stevens,[5] 1986	ICLH	19	RA (19)	4.5 y	83
Bolton-Maggs et al,[6] 1985	ICLH	62	RA (34), OA (13), SA (15)	5.5 y	47
Unger et al,[56] 1988	Mayo	23	RA (23)	5.6 y	65
Takakura et al,[57] 1990	Takakura cemented	33	OA (20), RA (11), SA (2)	8.8 y (metal), 6.7 y (ceramic)	15
Kofoed,[58] 2004	Cylindrical 2-piece cemented	28	RA (13), OA (15)	12 y	70

Abbreviations: OA, osteoarthritis; RA, rheumatoid arthritis; SA, Traumatic arthritis. None of the ankles considered by the FDA in their ankle classification was successful and all have been abandoned.

Data from Buechel FF, Pappas MJ. Principles of human joint replacement—design and clinical application. Berlin Heidelberg: Springer Verlag; 2011:116.

Neufeld and Lee[59] also state, "Several reasons for the long-term failure of the early prostheses have been suggested. First, many original designs required excessive bone resections and relied on cement fixation onto soft cancellous bone. Constrained prostheses placed excessive stress on the cement-cancellous bone interface. Subsequently the main reason for their failure was aseptic loosening. Unconstrained prostheses...failure occurred due to malleolar and soft-tissue impingement...Therefore, the failure of early designs may have been caused by the lack of respect for the anatomy, kinematics, alignment and stability of the ankle joint."

Furthermore, they state, "They (early constrained designs) have failed to incorporate the biomechanical characteristics of the ankle joint...The design of the implant should permit effective transfer of joint loads, be inherently stable, allow ease of surgical implantation/removal with minimum bone loss, and have resistance to wear, creep, fatigue failure and compressive shear loading."[59]

Therefore, despite encouraging early results, long-term studies proved that these ankle devices were not viable and were subsequently abandoned by the orthopedic community in favor of arthrodesis.

FIRST-GENERATION MOBILE-BEARING TOTAL ANKLES

In **Tables 2** and **3**, it may be seen that both the early LCS, B-P and STAR ankle performances, although not equal to the acceptance standard for hips and knees, are superior in performance to ankle fusion and, therefore, could be considered acceptable devices.

Analysis

STAR
Of the first-generation mobile-bearing designs, the STAR has the best clinical performance. Furthermore, this device provides essentially normal gait.[58] This good performance is further evidenced by the premarket approval, based on a well-controlled clinical trial by the FDA, allowing, for the first time, the sale of a mobile-bearing ankle in the United Stated of America.[66]

The primary fault of the STAR, however, is that it loses congruity in the event of inversion or eversion.

The B-P Mark I (LCS)
The LCS design, although performing well in the short term, experienced degradation in performance with time. The most frequent cause of failure is related to talar subsidence. This subsidence was due to several causes. The long fin allowed distal fixation to occur, leading the stress protection of the proximal talus. This contributed to atrophy and collapse of the talus, leading to talar component subsidence and bearing extrusion and wear.

In examining the blood supply to the talus,[67] it was concluded that the long central fin may be disrupting blood supply excessively, further contributing to talar necrosis and collapse. This evauation and others led to the development of the current B-P Mark III ankle.

ANKLE REPLACEMENTS AVAILABLE IN THE UNITED STATES
FDA-Cleared Fixed-Bearing Devices

These devices, the Inbone, Salto, and Agility ankles, have been cleared (not approved) for sale in the United States because they were found to be the substantial equivalent of those devices used by the FDA to establish the classification for such clearance.

Table 2
Long-term results of the LCS and B-P ankles

	Buechel et al,[17] 2004	Buechel and Pappas,[61] 1988	Keblish PA et al, unpublished data, 1990	Doets,[14] 2002	Doets et al,[62] 2006	San Giovanni et al,[16] 2006
Number of cases	40 (38 Patients)	23	237	58	30 (28 Patients)	21
M/F	Male = 20 Female = 20	Male = 12 Female = 11			Male = 2 Female = 26	
Age (mean)	55	56	57	55	56	—
Diagnosis	PTA = 21 (52.5%) OA = 7 (17.5%) RA = 9 (22%) Fusion = 3 (7.5%)	PTA = 10 (43.5%) OA = 4 (17.4%) RA = 6 (26.1%) AVN = 2 (8.7%) Fusion = 1 (4.3%)	PTA, OA, RA	RA, JCA, PA	RA = 25 (88%) JCA = 1 (4%) PA = 1 (4%) OA = 1 (4%)	RA
Follow-up	Mean 10 y (2–20 y)	Mean 35 mo (24–64 mo)	Mean 45 mo (18–72 mo)	Avg 6 y (2–13 y)	Avg 6 y (3–9 y)	Mean 5.5 y (3.3–9.0 y)
Delayed wound healing	9 (23%)	4 (19%)	2 (1%)	0 (0%)	3 (10%)	—
Talar subsidence	6 (15%)	0 (0%)	3 (2%)	0 (0%)	0 (0%)	2 (10%)
Bearing subluxation	4 (10%)	1 (5%)	11 (5%)	0 (0%)	3 (10%)	0 (0%)
Severe bearing wear	4 (10%)	0 (0%)	17 (7%)	2 (3%)	0 (0%)	1 (5%)
Malleolar fracture	3 (8%)	1 (5%)	6 (11%)	—	5 (17%)	—
Infection	2 (5%)	1 (5%)	9 (4%)	1 (2%)	1 (3%)	2 (10%)
Reflex sympathic dystrophy	2 (5%)	2 (10%)	1 (1%)	0 (0%)	0 (0%)	—
Varus/valgus deformity	—	—	—	6 (10%)	—	—
Tibial loosening	0 (0%)	0 (0%)	6 (3%)	3 (5%)	1 (3%)	1 (5%)
Survivorship (percentage)	74.2 (Kaplan-Meier) revision for any reason at 20 y	100 (Kaplan-Meier) revision for any reason at 5 y	90.7 (Kaplan-Meier) revision for any reason at 6 y	—	—	—
Average overall clinical score (percentage)	70 (NJOHAEF)	83.7 (NJOHAEF)	81.5 (NJOHAEF)	74 (NJOHAEF)	84 (NJOHAEF)	87 (AOFAS)

Abbreviations: PTA, post-traumatic arthritis; AVN, avascular necrosis; JCA, Juvenile arthritis; NJOHAEF, New Jersey Hospital Ankle Evaluation Form; AOFAS, Orthopaedic Foot and Ankle Society ankle score, OA, osteoarthritis; RA, rheumatoid arthritis; SA, Traumatic arthritis.

Data from Buechel FF, Pappas MJ. Principles of human joint replacement—design and clinical application. Berlin Heidelberg: Springer Verlag; 2011:121.

Table 3
Long-term results of the STAR ankle

Study	Valderrabano et al,[13] 2004	Schernberg[63] 1998	Kofoed and Sorensen,[64] 1988	Kofoed and Danborg,[65] 1995
Device	STAR Mobile Bearing TAR	STAR mobile-bearing TAR	STAR mobile-bearing TAR	STAR mobile-bearing TAR
Number of cases	68 (65 Patients)	131	Cemented = 33 Cementless = 25 Total 58	76
M/F	Male = 31 (48%) Female = 34 (52%)		Male cemented = 14 Female cemented = 19 Male cementless = 16 Female cementless = 9	Male = 35 (46%) Female = 41 (54%)
Age (mean)	56	—	Cemented = 60 Cementless = 58	56
Diagnosis	PTA = 48 (71%) RA = 11 (16%) OA = 9 (13%)	OA, RA	Cemented RA = 13 Cemented OA = 20 Cementless RA = 3 Cementless OA = 22	OA = 44 (58%), RA = 22 (29%), PA = 4 (6%), AVN = 4 (6%), failed fusion = 1 (1%)
Follow-up	Mean 3.7 y (2.4–6.2 y)	6 y	Cemented = 9.3 ± 2.7 Cementless = 9.5 ± 1.7	10 y
Delayed wound healing	—	—	—	—
Talar subsidence	1 (4%)	—	—	—
Bearing subluxation	1 (4%)	—	—	—
Severe bearing wear	3 (13%)	—	Cementless 1 (2%)	—
Malleolar fracture	0 (0%)	—	—	—
Infection	0 (0%)	—	—	—
Reflex sympathic dystrophy	1 (6%)	—	Cemented 1 (2%)	—
Tibial component loosening	2 (9%)	—	Cemented 6 (10%) Cementless 1 (2%)	—
Survivorship (%)	87 (After component related revision) at 6 y	87.3 (Kofoed, 1986) at 6 y	70 Cemented 95 Cementless (revision/ removal for any reason) at 9 y	86.7 (Kofoed, 1986) (revision for any reason) at 10 y
Average clinical score overall (percentage)	85 (AOFAS)	85 (Kofoed, 1986)	Cemented = 74.2 ± 19.3 Cementless = 91.9 ± 7.4	—

Data from Buechel FF, Pappas MJ. Principles of human joint replacement—design and clinical application. Berlin Heidelberg: Springer Verlag; 2011:chapter 4.

Unfortunately, in the case of ankle devices, such a designation provides only a negative connotation because all of the devices used for this purpose were later found to be failures and withdrawn from the market. Thus, the fact that they can be sold does not imply that it is safe to do so, but because they are substantially equivalent to failed devices, a more reasonable inference is that they are not safe. The comments of Neufeld and Lee[59] apply to these devices as well as those used for the FDA classification. Furthermore, all of these devices suffer from serious, fundamental, design defects-excessive contact stresses and/or constraints.

There are no published clinical data on the Inbone and Salto devices. The data on the Agility are extensive but generally negative, as described by Buechel and Pappas.[11] Thus, none of these devices seems appropriate as an alternative to fusion because they are unproved devices of a failed type with serious design flaws.

The Inbone ankle replacement

This design has other weaknesses in addition to the general defects of fixed-bearing devices (ie, excessive constraint and/or contact pressures); these are

1. Excessive bone resection. As seen in **Fig. 10**, the entire dome of the talus is resected, weakening it materially. Furthermore, the large diameter talar component fixation peg substantially interferes with the talar blood supply.
2. The complex tibial stem is unnecessary.[17,61] The Inbone stem increases cost, complicates implantation, and introduces the possibility of micromotion between the assembled elements and, thus, reactive metallic wear particles. The argument made by Wright Medical Technologies[68] that ankles suffer from problems of tibial fixation due to lack of long stems and tibial windows[66] is not supported by any evidence and is, in any event, untrue in light of the successful use of windows and short stems by the B-P ankle. Talar fixation is the most significant complication, not tibial fixation.[14,62]

The further argument used by Wright[68] to justify its use of a thick, fixed bearing is nonsense and is discussed previously and by Buechel and Pappas.[46] Furthermore,

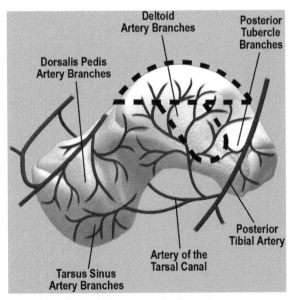

Fig. 10. Excessive talar resection and blood supply disruption.

the argument that precision of implantation can overcome all the problems of overconstraint and excessive contact stress is invalid and not supported by the references they cite. Wright sold only the mobile-bearing B-P ankle while it was available to them.

The Salto Talaris ankle replacement

The Salto Talaris ankle replacement is an FDA-dictated, fixed-bearing version of the mobile-bearing device sold outside the United States. Again there is unnecessary resection and interruption of the talar blood supply but not to the extent of the Inbone. Similarly, Tornier uses the same unsupported and irrational rationale that precision in implant placement can substitute for overconstraint and for incongruity. If Tornier believed that was the case, they would be selling the fixed-bearing version in Europe rather than their mobile-bearing version.

The Agility ankle replacement

The Agility is approximately 3 decades old. Due to its poor performance,[11] a series of modifications has been made to attempt to overcome various design defects. The latest iteration, the Agility LP, seems to offer some improvement but the fundamental problems of excessive bone resection, overconstraint, and excessive contact stress remain. The design is so new that no useful clinical data on its performance are yet available.

DePuy only sells its mobile-bearing Mobility ankle in Europe.

FDA-Approved Mobile-Bearing Ankle Replacement

The only approved ankle device is the STAR, which was finally approved in 2009 after a 2-year noninferiority with respect to fusion study.[69,70] Saltzman and colleagues[66] report the results of a study of 158 patients (from 10 centers) who had ankle replacement and 66 patients (in 5 different centers) who had fusion. In addition, they report the results of a 435-patient FDA-monitored continued access study of the STAR arthroplasty.

Based on these studies, particularly the continued access study where improved instrumentation was used, at least in the short term, STAR arthroplasty is superior to arthrodesis. Coupled with the results of the STAR (shown in **Table 3**), which show superiority to fusion in the midterm and long term, the STAR seems preferable to fusion.

THE FUTURE

The STAR, although superior to fusion, does not approach the performance of well-designed hip, knee, or even ankle devices. Fortunately, the evolution of the B-P ankle design has advanced to the point where a device comparable in performance to the hip and knee is possible.[17,69] Although the clinical results of the latest B-P ankle meet the acceptance criteria for hips and knees described previously, an unexpected problem of cyst formation leading to talar and even tibial component subsidence has been observed.[50] Although wear in the bearing is extremely low, even minor wear can produce such cysts.

A solution involving better polishing of the talar component and more wear-resistant highly cross-linked UHMWPE is now under trial with initially promising results. Hopefully, ankle replacements comparable to well-designed hip and knee replacements will become available in the near future in the United States as they are now in Europe, where almost all ankle replacements are of the mobile-bearing type.

SUMMARY

FDA clearance of an ankle device does not imply safety because the FDA classification of class II for ankles finds that such ankles are substantially equivalent to the devices found to be failures. All of the FDA-cleared fixed-bearing devices can, therefore, not be considered acceptable. All such devices available in the United States fail to satisfy reasonable design criteria because they all have serious design defects. Furthermore, none has acceptable, published clinical performance data. Thus, these designs should not be considered for clinical use.

Only the STAR, which has reasonable midterm and long-term results and FDA approval, seems preferable to fusion and acceptable for ankle reconstruction. Still better devices are on the horizon.

REFERENCES

1. Jensen NC, Kroner K. Total ankle joint replacement: a clinical follow up. Orthopedics 1992;15(2):236–9.
2. Kitaoka HB, Patzer GL. Clinical results of the Mayo total ankle arthroplasty. J Bone Joint Surg Am 1996;78(11):1658–64.
3. Kitaoka HB, Patzer GL, Ilstrup DM, et al. Survivorship analysis of the mayo total ankle arthroplasty. J Bone Joint Surg Am 1994;76:974–9.
4. Wynn AH, Wilde AH. Long-term follow-up of conaxial (beck-stefee) total ankle arthroplasty. Foot Ankle 1992;13:303–6.
5. Helm R, Stevens J. Long-term results of total ankle replacement. J Arthroplasty 1986;1(4):271–7.
6. Bolton-Maggs BG, Sudlow RA, Freeman MA. Total ankle arthroplasty. A long-term review of the London Hospital experience. J Bone Joint Surg Br 1985;67(5):785–90.
7. SooHoo NF, Zingmond DS, Ko CY. Comparison of reoperation rates following ankle arthrodesis and total ankle arthroplasty. J Bone Joint Surg Am 2007;89(10):243–9.
8. Krause FG, Windolf M, Bora B, et al. Impact of complications in total ankle and ankle arthrodesis analyzed with a validated outcomes measurement. J Bone Joint Surg Am 2011;93(9):830–9.
9. Coester LM, Salzman CJ, Leupold J, et al. Long-term results following ankle arthrodesis for post traumatic arthritis. J Bone Joint Surg Am 2001;83(2):219–28.
10. Federal Register (1982) Section 888.3110: 47/128:29070.
11. Buechel FF, Pappas MJ. Principles of human joint replacement—design and clinical application. Springer Verlag, Berlin, Heidelberg; 2011. chapter 4:108-118.
12. AOFS announces results of clinical trials with the Star ankle replacement device. Available at: www. News-medical.net/2009826/AOFS-announces-results-of-clinical-trials. Accessed March 3, 2012.
13. Valderrabano V, Hintermann B, Dick W. Scandinavian total ankle replacement. Clinical Orthop 2004;424:47–56.
14. Doets HC. 2–13 Year results with the LCS/Buechel-Pappas Mobile Bearing Prosthesis. ERASS; 2002.
15. Su EP, Kahn B, Figgie MP. Total ankle replacement in patients with rheumatoid arthritis. Clinical Orthop 2004;424:32–8.
16. San Giovanni T, Keblish DJ, Thomas WH, et al. Eight year results of a minimally constrained total ankle arthroplasty. Foot Ankle Int 2006;27:418–26.
17. Buechel FF, Buechel FF Jr, Pappas MJ. Twenty year evaluation of cementless mobile-bearing total ankle replacement. Clinical Orthop 2004;424:19–26.
18. Leardini A, O'Connor JJ, Catani F, et al. Mobility of the human ankle and the design of total ankle replacement. Clinical Orthop 2004;424:39–46.
19. Leardini A, O'Connor JJ, Catani F, et al. Kinematics of the human ankle complex in passive motion; a single degree of freedom system. J Biomech 1999;32:111–8.

20. Stauffer RN, Chao EY, Brewster RC. Force and motion analysis of the normal, diseased and prosthetic ankle joint. Transactions of the proceedings of the 23rd Annual Meeting of the ORS. Las Vegas (NV): 44. 1977.
21. Fitzgerald E, Chao EY, Hoffman RE. Goniometric measurement of ankle motion A method for clinical evaluation. Transactions of the proceedings of the 23rd Annual Meeting of the ORS. Las Vegas (NV): 43. 1977.
22. Stauffer RN, Chao EY. Torsional stability of the Mayo total ankle arthroplasty. Transactions of the proceedings of the 25th Annual Meeting of the ORS. San Francisco (CA): 112. 1979.
23. Harris EC. Elements of structural engineering. New York: Roland Donald Press; 1954.
24. Ludema KC. Wear. ASM Handbook, Volume 18, Friction, Lubrication, and wear Technology, The American Society of Materials; 1992. p. 175–280.
25. Amenzade YA. Theory of elasticity. Moscow (Russia): Mir; 1979.
26. Black J. Biological performance of materials—fundamentals of biocompatibility. New York: Marcel Dekker; 1981.
27. Hutton DV. Fundamentals of finite element analysis. New York: McGraw-Hill; 2004.
28. Lawallen DG, Rand JA. Failure of metal-baked patellar components after total knee arthroplasty. Knee 1993;2:37–41.
29. Takeuchi T, Lathi VJ, Khan AM, et al. Patellofemoral contact pressures exceed the compressive yield strength of UHMWPE in total knee arthroplasties. J Arthroplasty 1995;10:363–8.
30. Wright TM, Bartel, DL. The problem of surface damage in polyethylene total knee components. Clinical Orthopaedics and Related Research 1986;205:67–74.
31. Engh GA, Dwyer KA, Hannes CK. Polyethylene wear of metal-backed tibial components in total and unicompartmental knee prostheses. J Bone Joint Surg Br 1992;74(1):9–17.
32. Rose RM, Goldfarb EV, Ellis E, et al. On pressure dependence of the wear of ultra-high molecular weight polyethylene. Wear 1983;92:99–111.
33. Bartel DL, Rawlinson J, Burstein A, et al. Stresses in polyethylene components of contemporary total knee replacements. Clinical Orthopaedics 1995;317: 76–82.
34. Bartel DL, Bicknell VL, Wright TM. The effect of conformity, thickness and material on stresses in ultra-high molecular weight polyethylene components for total joint replacement. J Bone Joint Surg Am 1986;68:1041.
35. Pappas MJ, Makris G, Buechel FF. Evaluation of contact stress in metal plastic knee replacements. In: Pizzoferrato A, et al, editors. Biomaterials and clinical applications. Amsterdam: Elsevier; 1897. p. 259–64 Clemson SC:101.
36. Pappas MJ, Buechel FF. New Jersey knee simulator. Proceedings of the Eleventh International Biomaterials Symposium held at Clemson (SC): 1979. p. 101.
37. Bartell DL, Wright TM, Edwards DL. The effect of metal backing on stresses in polyethylene acetabular components. The hip: proceedings of Hip Society:229. St Louis (MO): CV Mosby; 1983.
38. Willert HG, Semlitsh M. Reaction of the articular capsule to wear products of artificial joint prostheses. J Biomed Mater Res 1977;11:134–64.
39. Gelante JO, Lamons J, Spector M, et al. The biological effects of implant materials. J Orthop Res 1991;9:760–75.
40. Dowson D, ElHady Diab MM, Gilles BJ, et al. Influence of counterface topography on the wear of UHMWPE under wet and dry conditions. In: Lee HL, editor. The Proceedings of the American Chemical Society, Polymer Wear and its Control, ACS Symp, vol. 287. Ser; 1885. p. 171–87.

41. Pappas MJ. Makris G, Buechel FF. Comparison of Wear Of UHMWPe Cups Articulating With Co-Cr and TiN Coated Femoral Heads. Transactions of the Society of Biomaterials XIII:36. 1990.

42. Seely FB, Smith JO. Advanced mechanics of materials. Chapter 14. New York: Wiley and Sons; 1958.

43. Pappas MJ, Makris G, Buechel FF. Contact stresses in metal—plastic total knee replacements: a theoretical and experimental study. Biomedical engineering technical report. South Orange (NJ): Biomedical Engineering Trust; 1986.

44. Hostalen GU. Hoechst Aktiengesellschaft, Verkauf Kunstoffe, 6230 Frankfurt am Main 80:22. 1982.

45. Pappas MJ, Makris G, Buechel FF. Wear in prosthetic knee joints. Scientific Exhibit, 59th Annual Meeting of the AAOS, Washington, DC: 1992.

46. Buechel FF, Pappas MJ. Principles of human joint replacement—design and clinical application. Springer Verlag, Berlin Heidelberg; 2011. chapter 2:66-72.

47. Van Loon CJM, HU HP, Van Horn JR, et al. The Geomedic prosthesis - A long term follow-up study. Acta Orthopaedica Belgica 1993;59(1):40–4.

48. Moyad TF, Thornhill T, Estok D. Evaluation and management of the infected total hip and knee. Orthopedics 2008;31(6):581–8.

49. Buechel FF, Buechel FF Jr, Pappas MJ. Ten-year evaluation of cementless meniscal bearing total ankle replacement. Foot Ankle Int 2003;24(6):462–72.

50. Buechel FF. Osteolysis after total ankle replacement presented at the 35th annual orthopaedic surgeon & trauma society meeting. Netherlands Antilles: Bonaire; 2009.

51. Buechel FF, Pappas MJ, Greenwald AS. Use of survivorship and contact stress analysis to predict the long-term efficacy of new generation joint replacement designs—a model for FDA device evaluation. Orthop Rev 1991;20(1):50–5.

52. Buchner M, Sabo D. Ankle fusion attributable to posttraumatic arthritis: a long-term follow-up of 48 patients. Clin Orthop Relat Res 2003;(406):155–64.

53. Stauffer RN. Total joint arthroplasty. The ankle. Mayo Clin Proc 1979;54(9):570–5.

54. Scholz KC. Total ankle arthroplasty using biological fixation components compared to ankle arthrodesis. Orthopedics 1987;10(1):125–31.

55. Waugh TR, Evanski PM, McMaster WC. Irvine ankle arthroplasty. Prosthetic design and surgical technique. Clin Orthop 1976;(114):180–4.

56. Unger AS, Inglis AE, Mow CS, et al. Total ankle arthroplasty in rheumatoid arthritis: a long-term follow-up study. Foot Ankle 1988;8(4):173–9.

57. Takakura Y, Tanaka Y, Sugimoto K, et al. Ankle arthroplasty. A comparative study of cemented metal and uncemented ceramic prostheses. Clin Orthop 1990; 1(252):209–16.

58. Kofoed H. Scandinavian Total Ankle Replacement (STAR). Clinical Orthop 2004; 424:73–9.

59. Neufeld SK, Lee TH. Total ankle arthroplasty: indications, results, and biomechanical rationale. Am J Orthop (Belle Mead NJ) 2000;29(8):593–602.

60. Lachiewicz PF, Inglis AE, Ranawat CS. Total ankle replacement in rheumatoid arthritis. J Bone Joint Surg Am 1984;66(3):340–3.

61. Buechel FF, Pappas MJ. The new jersey low-contact stress ankle replacement system: biomechanical rationale and review of the first 23 cementless cases. Foot Ankle 1988;8(8):279–90.

62. Doets HC, et al. Total ankle arthroplasty in inflammatory joint desease. J Bone Joint Surg Am 2006;86:1272–86.

63. Schernberg F. Current results of ankle arthroplasty—European multi-center study of cementless ankle arthroplasty. Chapter 9. In: Kofoed H, editor. Current status of ankle arthroplasty. Berlin: Springer; 1998.

64. Kofoed H, Sorensen TS. Ankle arthroplasty for rheumatoid arthritis and osteoarthritis: prospective long-term study of cemented replacements. J Bone Joint Surg Br 1998;80(2):328–32.
65. Kofoed H, Danborg L. Biological fixation of ankle arthroplasty. Foot 1995;5(1):27–31.
66. Saltzmen CL, Mann RA, Ahrens JE, et al. Prospective controlled trial of STAR total ankle replacement versus ankle fusion: initial results. Foot Ankle Int 2009;30(7): 579–96.
67. Mulfiner GL, Trueta J. The blood supply of the talus. J Bone Joint Surg Am 1970; 52(1):160–7.
68. Inbone Total Ankle system, Sugical Technique. Wright Medical Technologies; chapter 1;7. 2009.
69. U.S. Food and Drug Administration. STRA Ankle Premarket Approval Panel Meeting Presentation 4-24-2007. Available at: http://www/fda/ohrms/dockets/ac/07/slides/2007-4299s1-01.pdf. Accessed March 30, 2012.
70. Doets HC, Brand R, Nelissen RG. Total ankle arthroplasty in infalamitory joint desiese with the use of two mobile-bearing designs. J Bone Joint Surg Am 2006;88(6):1272–84.

Periprosthetic Aseptic Osteolysis in Total Ankle Replacement
Cause and Management

Mark T.R. Gaden, MBBS, BMedSci, MRCS,
Benjamin J. Ollivere, MBBS, BA (Oxon), MRCS (Trauma & Orthopaedics)*

KEYWORDS

- Aseptic loosening • Ankle • Arthroplasty • Osteolysis • Revision arthroplasty

KEY POINTS

- Osteolysis is the major cause of failure of total ankle replacement, the failure rate increases with time and results in loss of fixation of the prosthesis.
- The osteolytic process is driven by phagocytosable wear debris and is initiated by macrophage activation. The activation of macrophages results in the initiation of a biologic cascade and the final common pathway of activation of RANK by RANK-L and osteoclast-mediated loss of bone.
- Bone loss prevents a difficult problem for revision ankle replacement that may be addressed through bone grafting or custom prosthesis. Bone grafting may be used to restore bone stock, whereas custom (or stemmed) prosthesis may maximize fixation in cases with severe bone loss.
- Further clinical work is required to evaluate treatments for periprosthetic aseptic osteolysis in total ankle replacement.

BACKGROUND

Osteolysis is the loss of bone secondary to a pathologic process. With relation to joint replacements of any type, osteolysis is the term given to periprosthetic bone loss following implant arthroplasty.

Although reports of the outcomes of ankle replacements are scarce within the scientific literature and the pathophysiology of failure mechanisms is unclear, there is evidence implicating osteolytic changes as one of the main drivers of ankle implant failure and revision surgery.[1–3] In 2011, the Scandinavian ankle replacement registry reported on 780 primary ankle replacements with an overall failure rate of 31% at

Division of Orthopaedic & Accident Surgery, Nottingham University Hospital NHS Trust, Derby Road, Nottingham NG7 2UH, UK
* Corresponding author.
E-mail address: Ben.Ollivere@nuh.nhs.uk

Clin Podiatr Med Surg 30 (2013) 145–155
http://dx.doi.org/10.1016/j.cpm.2012.10.006   podiatric.theclinics.com

10-years.[1] Of the 168 ankle revisions recorded on Swedish total ankle replacement registry, 67 were revised for aseptic loosening, the leading cause of revision.

The loss of bone from the periprosthetic region can result in loss of fixation and eventual subsidence, loosening, and migration of either or both components. In a systematic review including 1,105 total ankle replacements, Gougoulias and colleagues[4] recorded a 30.2% incidence of radiolucencies and 10% rate of subsidence or migration in surviving total ankle replacement at a mean of 5-years follow-up.

The natural history of total joint arthroplasty is of an increasing rate of failure as the interval from implantation increases. The mode of failure, however, changes over time. During the first few years after implantation, early infection and surgical error predominate. However, as time progresses, aseptic loosening predominate as the primary modes of failure in all forms of arthroplasty. The results for each joint and prosthesis differ and the success rates are measured as absolute survival at a 5-year or 10-year benchmark or, most commonly, using a Kaplan-Meier survival analysis model.[1–3]

It has become commonplace to revise failed total hip and knee replacements to revision components, thereby maintaining function. However, only 62% of 108 revisions reported by Gougoulias and colleagues[4] were revised to revision prosthesis. This highlights the need to improve treatment and revision of aseptic osteolysis in total ankle replacements. The understanding and treatment of the osteolytic process in general, and specifically in the ankle, is key to improving survivorship and providing viable surgical revision alternatives.

DEFINING OSTEOLYSIS

Aseptic loosening is a process in which, in the absence of infection, the interface between the prosthesis and the bone loses fixation and the prosthesis fails. The most widely accepted explanation for this is that the generation of particulate debris from a prosthesis results in an inflammatory response leading to bone resorption or osteolysis.[5] Failure due to aseptic loosening of one or both of the components of all types of joint replacement is the most common reason for revision surgery.

Although there is general agreement that aseptic loosening is due to the production of wear debris from the joint articulation, this is where the consensus of opinion ends. There is no clear, agreed on definition of aseptic loosening. Furthermore, there is variability in the outcome and revision rates within published groups of patients implanted with the same prosthesis, even within the same hospital. Objective scientific study into the causative factors, natural history, and incidence of this condition is, therefore, difficult.

THE PROCESS OF ASEPTIC LOOSENING

It was originally described by Wolff[6] that bone responds to and remodels with mechanical forces. Mechanical loading of bone can cause remodeling and compensatory growth.[7] There are widespread reports in the hip arthroplasty literature of proximal femoral resorption with distally fixing prostheses and it is likely that this stress shielding is in part responsible for the characteristic patterns of loosening described by Gruen and colleagues.[8] Forces pass from the pelvis through the stem of the femoral component and into the distal femur, bypassing the proximal femora. The subsequent stress shielding of the proximal femora results in bone loss and the characteristic failure pattern of "cantilever bending"[8] associated with distally fixed prostheses. There is little clinical study of the stress-shielding effects of different models of ankle prosthesis, Bouguecha and colleagues[9] have performed a comprehensive finite element analysis model that suggests it is reasonable to assume the same strain-adaptive bone remodeling process occurs in the same manner as in total hip arthroplasty.

It is important to distinguish this form of mechanical loosening, which is a function of failure to load the proximal femora, from the process of osteolysis, which is an active process and is a biologic response to wear debris.[10–12] Both result in a common mode of failure through loss of fixation and stem stability but through very different processes. In clinical practice the two often coexist.

THE PROCESS OF OSTEOLYSIS

The components of any prosthesis are either cemented into place with antibiotic impregnated polymethylmethacrylate, or implanted with uncemented fixation techniques. Modern designs of total ankle replacement rely on either bone ongrowth or bone ingrowth to the bone-prosthesis interface through use of porous coatings that provides a "biologic fixation." This eliminates the problems associated with wear debris from cement that have long (and often incorrectly) been associated with aseptic loosening in hip replacements. The earliest descriptions of osteolysis were following revision of cemented total hip replacements. Areas of bone loss and osteolysis were found in association with large granulomas filled with polymethylmethacrylate particles[13] and the incorrect association was made between the cement and osteolysis.

It is now commonly accepted that mechanical wear of the articulating surface releases particulate debris, although there have been some alternate explanations, including loss of bone due to increased fluid pressure.[10] This is phagocytosed, activating the macrophages and osteoclasts, and resulting in bone resorption. This mechanism and the existence of an underlying biologic process of aseptic osteolysis were first hypothesized by Willert and Semlitsch[11] in 1977. Osteolysis is an active biologic process that results in the loss of bone as a direct response to stimulation of macrophages by biologically active particles. Aseptic loosening is also closely associated with osteolysis, an active process of bone destruction and loss that is cell-mediated.[12]

Although originally described as "cement disease,"[11,13] it is now understood that any particulate debris may result in an osteolytic reaction. Ultrahigh molecular weight polyethylene (UHMWPE), polymethylmethacrylate cement, Co-Cr, $Ti2O_3$, ZrO_2 particles have all been extensively shown to produce biologically active wear debris.[12]

GENERATION OF WEAR DEBRIS

The generation of wear particles occurs at the two primary articulating surfaces of the tibial component and talar component against the UHMWPE component; mainly through adhesive wear.[14] These biologically active particles form most of the burden of wear debris in total ankle replacement, although metal ions and polymethylmethacrylate particles have also been identified in hip and knee replacements, it seems unlikely this plays a major role in loosening of total ankle replacement.

The size and morphology of particulate wear debris has a profound effect on their biologic activity. Most UHMWPE wear particles are submicron (<1 μm) in size. This makes visualization with light microscopy difficult due to the wavelength of visible light (0.4–0.7-μm). This led to an initial underestimation of the number and volume of particles in periprosthetic tissues. The use of proteolytic enzymes on periprosthetic tissues, and subsequent density-gradient centrifugation,[15] has allowed accurate characterization of smaller particle numbers and size by use of a particle analyzer. Electron microscopy studies have confirmed that most wear debris particles are submicron in size, with 70% to 90% of UHMWPE particles measuring approximately 0.5-μm.[15]

The biologic effects of wear debris vary with particulate size and number:

- Phagocytosable particles (<10 mm) are more biologically active
- At high concentrations, particulate debris becomes cytotoxic and provokes apoptosis in the macrophage.
- Phagocytosis results release of tumor necrosis factor alpha (TNF-α), which larger particles do not evoke.[16]
- Metal, UHMWPE, and ceramic wear debris provoke a similar response.[12]
- Activity of UHMWPE debris is size- and concentration-dependent.[17,18]

EFFECT OF WEAR DEBRIS

An active biologic cascade resulting in the activation of osteoclasts and loss of bone occurs as a direct response to particulate wear debris. There is no currently universally consensus as to the precise mechanism, precipitating factors, and regulatory factors of this cascade. Instead, there are many studies examining the process from different perspectives.

Histopathological studies have shown profuse macrophage infiltration into periprosthetic tissues and the interstitial membrane.[11] In addition, polarized light microscopy studies have identified large volumes of periprosthetic UHMWPE debris undergoing phagocytosis. There is histopathological evidence for involvement of macrophages, osteoblasts, osteoclasts, fibroblasts, and other antigen-presenting cells, which have all been implicated in osteolysis. The role of each is briefly outlined below:

Macrophages
- Activation of a macrophage-mediated response is central to the initiation of an osteolytic response[19]
- Macrophages phagocytose all types of wear debris and production of proinflammatory signal molecules[20]
- Activated macrophages secrete cytokines, including prostaglandin E2, TNF-α,[21] interleukin (IL) 1-beta and IL6[22]
- Activation of macrophages also alters expression of matrix regulatory proteins, including matrix metalloproteinases.[23]

Exposure of macrophages to particulate wear debris is the critical initiating event in osteolysis.

Osteoblasts
- Osteoblast inhibition may result in bone loss[19]
- Lohmann and colleagues[24] established that osteoblasts phagocytose wear debris, modulating cytokine expression in cultured osteoblasts.
- Exposure of osteoblasts to UHMWPE reduces collagen type I and III production[25] and inhibit osteoblast differentiation.[26]

Current data are far from conclusive but do implicate regulation of osteoblast activity and differentiation in osteolysis.

Osteoclasts
- Osteoclasts are the only cell lineage capable of active bone resorption[27]
- Osteoclasts infiltrate tissue surrounding loose implants[28]
- Monocyte chemotactic protein-1 and macrophage inflammatory protein-1a recruit osteoclasts from precursor cells and expression is increased surrounding periprosthetic tissues[29]
- Activation of osteoclasts is via signal pathways from activated macrophages, including IL1, TNF-α, and IL6.

Osteoclasts are responsible for the active removal of bone as a response to wear debris and are the final common target for several interacting pathways in the osteolytic cascade.

Receptor activator of nuclear factor κ B and its ligand
- RANK receptor is a membrane receptor found on osteoclasts
- Ligand binding at this receptor is the initiator for osteoclast differentiation
- Osteoprotegerin is the antagonist for this pathway, is secreted by osteoblasts, and regulates osteoclast activity.[30]

Much emphasis has been placed on the importance of the receptor activator of nuclear factor κ B (RANK) and its ligand (RANK-L) in osteolysis.[30] The RANK pathway is a key modulator of bone turnover.[19] Alteration in ratio of RANK-L to osteoprotegerin is reflected in changes to the rate and type of bone turnover and, consequently, has been implicated in many metabolic diseases of bone.

CLASSIFICATION OF OSTEOLYTIC DEFECTS

Aseptic loosening is characterized by loss of fixation at the bone-cement or prosthesis-cement interfaces and is often associated with large osteolytic bone defects (**Fig. 1**). The American Academy of Orthopedic Surgeons classifies these as two distinct, but potentially related, entities.[31]

Although the American Academy of Orthopedic Surgeons classification relates specifically to hip and knee replacement, it is a useful guide to treatment and can be applied to total ankle replacement.

- Cavitatory defects have an intact cortical rim and, subsequently, may be treated with bone grafting, impaction grafting, or may be ignored. The structural integrity of the bone is not compromised.
- With segmental defects, the osteolytic lesion has resulted in loss of structural integrity of the cortex. Consequently, the bone is not able to support an implanted prosthesis without structural repair. Segmental defects can be bone grafted; however, for impaction grafting, a segmental defect must be converted to a cavitatory defect with the use of structural bone graft.
- Combined defects have a combination of the above pathologic conditions.

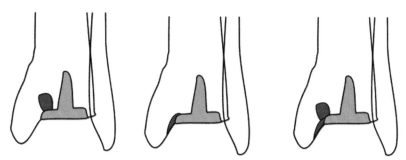

Cavitatory Defect   Segmental Defect   Combined Defect

Fig. 1. Anterior-posterior illustrations of the classification of osteolytic defects (from left to right) as cavitatory, segmental, and combined. The red represents the osteolytic defect about the tibial tray.

ZONES IN TOTAL ANKLE REPLACEMENT

The presence of osteolytic lines indicates potential loss of fixation in that the bond between the prosthesis and the bone has been lost. This is most closely studied in hips. The prosthesis is divided into recognized zones (Gruen and colleagues[8]). This helps with clinical record keeping and, within the hip, has been shown to predict loosening.[2]

There are several described systems for allocating zones to ankle replacements. The numbering patterns for the two most common tibial component designs are shown in **Fig. 2**.

Hodgkinson and colleagues[32] validated their own criteria against intraoperative findings of 200 acetabula and found 94% to be loose when a complete radiolucent line was present compared with only 7% with a radiolucent line in a single zone. Harris criteria for radiological loosening when applied to a 6-year radiograph were found by Ollivere and colleagues[2] to be predictive of revision by the 12-year follow-up.

Further work is required to develop and establish suitable radiographic criteria for failure of total ankle replacement. Early recognition of osteolysis and, particularly, progressive radiographic changes may prevent catastrophic failure and component migration or fracture.

EVIDENCE FOR OSTEOLYSIS IN TOTAL ANKLE REPLACEMENT

Owing to the low numbers of published studies, and much shorter follow-up and implantation rates, there is little literature on osteolysis in total ankle replacements and, consequently, data and studies for large joint arthroplasties and basic science studies have to be generalized to the ankle joint. However, there are several differences in ankle replacement and, because of the unique biomechanics and susceptibility to surgical malalignment, total ankle replacement carries a higher and slightly different burden of aseptic loosening.

Rodrigues and colleagues[33] reported radiographically evident osteolysis in 77% of their 21 ankle replacements at less than 4-years of follow-up. This finding is echoed by Koivu and colleagues[34] who identified a 50% rate of osteolysis at just over 2-years of follow-up in their series of total ankle replacements. In both cases, however, most patients were asymptomatic, which echoes findings in total hip arthroplasty.[2]

The American Academy of Orthopedic Surgeons described patterns of osteolytic lesions that are well documented in total ankle replacement. Koivu and colleagues[34]

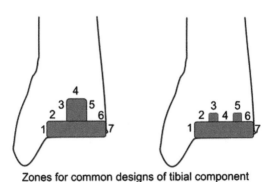

Zones for common designs of tibial component

Fig. 2. Anterior-posterior illustrations of the numeric order of zones for common designs of total ankle replacement tibial trays. These are important considerations for research collection on aseptic osteolysis.

reviewed 130 ankle replacements at the 6-year follow-up and identified 37% with osteolytic change. More than 20% of their patients demonstrated cavitatory osteolysis with cavities greater than 10 mm in size.

Although the major body of evidence for the osteolytic cascade comes from hip and tissue studies, it is not unreasonable to suppose that the pathways are identical. Koivu and colleagues[35] conducted an ex vivo study analyzing tissue from failed total ankle replacement, which confirmed the activation of the RANK to RANK-L pathway in failing total ankle joint replacements. They identified a similar foreign body response seen in other published studies, but were concerned that within the ankle joint necrotic autologous tissues may also be driving the macrophage response.

TREATMENT STRATEGIES

Broadly speaking, treatment of osteolytic and loose total ankle replacements can be divided into arthrodesis procedures (covered elsewhere in this issue) and strategies to revise the total ankle replacement while achieving restoration of bone stock or prosthesis stability fit without restoring bone stock. **Table 1** summarizes the different operative strategies to deal with bone defects.

Bone grafts have a range of biologic and structural properties and may be composed of autograft, allograft, xenograft, or artificial bone graft substitutes, the properties of bone grafts and substitutes are summarized in **Table 2**. The grafts can function to provide stability for prosthesis implantation (structural properties) or function to promote osseous repair and integration of the graft into the host bone (biologic properties). The choice of graft, surgical tactic, and type of grafting depends on the bone defect, choice of revision prosthesis or fusion, and the experience of the operating surgeon. Revision total ankle replacement with bone grafting should only be performed by surgeons experienced with complex primary and revision total ankle replacement surgery.

IMPACTION BONE GRAFTING

Impaction bone grafting is a technique for restoring bone stock in contained defects developed originally to address acetabular and femoral defects. The technique is only suitable for contained defects, meaning either cavitatory defects or other defects that have been contained through use of a mesh, augment, or structural graft. The

Table 1		
Bone defects and treatment options		
Defect Type	**Operative Strategy**	**Suitable Treatments**
Cavitatory	Restore bone stock	Impaction bone grafting Bone graft substitutes Allograft
	Achieve stability	Stemmed prosthesis Custom prosthesis
Segmental	Restore bone stock	Structural (cortical) graft Allograft
	Achieve stability	Stemmed prosthesis Custom prosthesis
Combined	Restore bone stock	Bulk allografting
	Achieve stability	Custom prosthesis

Table 2
Bone graft properties

Graft Type	Structural Properties	Biologic Activity	Osteoconductive Properties	Application
Cancellous autograft	+	++	+++	Impaction grafting Fusion
Cancellous allograft	+	+	++	Impaction grafting Fusion
Cortical autograft	+++	++	++	Structural grafting
Cortical allograft	+++	+	+	Structural grafting
Porous Ceramics (eg, hydroxyapatite)	++	−	+	Impaction grafting Fusion
Demineralized bone matrix	−	+++	−	Mix with other grafts to improve biology

technique of impaction grafting has been well described in hip and knee replacements. Lamberton and colleagues[36] described successful femoral impaction grafting in 540 hips with a 10-year survival of 98%. These results were echoed by Halliday and colleagues[37] who reported 226 patients with an impressive 99.1% survival at 10-years of follow-up.

BULK BONE GRAFTING

Several bulk bone grafting techniques are described in other areas of orthopedic surgery.[38] However, there are few reports of bulk bone grafting in revision total ankle replacement. Bulk bone grafting is a technique that involves bulk autograft or allograft applied with cables or screws to the recipient site. The incorporation of bulk bone graft involves creeping substitution and remodeling of the allograft into the bone by osteoclast-led cutting cones.

BYPASS WITH LONG STEM

Bypass of osteolytic lesions with longer stems is well described in hip and knee revision surgery. The revision prosthesis is implanted in the anatomic position, but the addition of stems (and/or wedges) allows the prosthesis to be placed on intact bone distal to the osteolytic lesion. When the prosthesis is loaded, the load passes through the prosthesis, along the stem, and into the distal bone. This provides initial fixation for the prosthesis but may offload or stress-shield the distal bone and result in further proximal bone loss.

This technique is particularly suited to segmental and combined defects, and has been used in revision total ankle replacement. Devries and colleagues[39] describe successful revision of failed Agility total ankle replacement systems (DePuy Orthopedics, Warsaw, IN, USA) to stemmed modular INBONE total ankle replacements (Wright Medical Technology, Inc, Memphis, TN, USA). In their series of five subjects, three revisions were successful at 12-months of follow-up.

An alternate approach is to augment or replace bone loss with a custom-designed prosthesis. There is little in the literature on the outcomes of such procedures in total ankle replacement, although Myerson and Won[40] and Ketz and colleagues[41] discuss the use of custom-designed prosthesis in revision total ankle replacements.

SUMMARY

There is precious little research into osteolysis within the setting of total ankle replacement. The process of osteolysis is well described in the basic science literature. However, it remains the largest limit to longevity in total ankle replacement. Application of surgical techniques developed in hip and knee replacement may allow for more revision surgery to succeed. Revision total ankle replacement surgery should only be performed by surgeons experienced with the complex techniques required for this form of surgery.

REFERENCES

1. Henricson A, Nilsson JA, Carlsson A. Ten-year survival of total ankle arthroplasties: a report on 780 cases from the Swedish Ankle Register. Acta Orthop 2011;82:655–9.
2. Ollivere B, Darrah C, Brankin RC, et al. The continued value of clinical and radiological surveillance: the Charnley Elite Plus hip replacement system at 12-years. J Bone Joint Surg Br 2009;91:720–4.
3. Porter M, Borrof M, Gregg P, et al. NJR annual report. UK National Joint Registry; 2012.
4. Gougoulias N, Khanna A, Maffulli N. How successful are current ankle replacements? A systematic review of the literature. Clin Orthop Relat Res 2010;468: 199–208.
5. Ollivere B, Wimhurst JA, Clark IM, et al. Current concepts in osteolysis. J Bone Joint Surg Br 2012;94:10–5.
6. Wolff J. Das Gesetz der Transformation der Knochen, Hirschwald, Berlin 1892.
7. Proff P, Romer P. The molecular mechanism behind bone remodelling: a review. Clin Oral Investig 2009;13:355–62.
8. Gruen TA, McNeice GM, Amstutz HC. Modes of failure of cemented stem-type femoral components: a radiographic analysis of loosening. Clin Orthop Relat Res 1979;141:17–27.
9. Bouguecha A, Weigel N, Behrens BA, et al. Numerical simulation of strain-adaptive bone remodelling in the ankle joint. Biomed Eng Online 2011;10:58.
10. Aspenberg P, van der Vis H. Fluid pressure may cause peri-prosthetic osteolysis: particles are not the only thing. Acta Orthop Scand 1998;69:1–4.
11. Willert HG, Semlitsch M. Reactions of the articular capsule to wear products of artificial joint prostheses. J Biomed Mater Res 1977;11:157–64.
12. Archibeck MJ, Jacobs JJ, Roebuck KA, et al. The basic science of peri-prosthetic osteolysis. Instr Course Lect 2001;50:185–95.
13. Jones LC, Hungerford DS. Cement disease. Clin Orthop Relat Res 1987;225: 192–206.
14. McKellop HA, Campbell P, Park SH, et al. The origin of submicron polyethylene wear debris in total hip arthroplasty. Clin Orthop Relat Res 1995;311:3–20.
15. Affatato S, Fernandes B, Tucci A, et al. Isolation and morphological characterisation of UHMWPE wear debris generated in vitro. Biomaterials 2001;22: 2325–31.
16. Horowitz SM, Doty SB, Lane JM, et al. Studies of the mechanism by which the mechanical failure of polymethylmethacrylate leads to bone resorption. J Bone Joint Surg Am 1993;75:802–13.
17. Catelas I, Petit A, Zukor DJ, et al. Induction of macrophage apoptosis by ceramic and polyethylene particles in vitro. Biomaterials 1999;20:625–30.

18. Catelas I, Huk OL, Petit A, et al. Flow cytometric analysis of macrophage response to ceramic and polyethylene particle: effects of size, concentration and composition. J Biomed Mater Res 1998;41:600–7.
19. Purdue PE, Koulouvaris P, Potter HG, et al. The cellular and molecular biology of peri-prosthetic osteolysis. Clin Orthop Relat Res 2007;454:251–61.
20. Nakashima Y, Sun DH, Trindade MC, et al. Signalling pathways for tumor necrosis factor-alpha and interleukin-6 expression in human macrophages exposed to titanium-alloy particulate debris in vitro. J Bone Joint Surg Am 1999;81:603–15.
21. Ingham E, Green TR, Stone MH, et al. Production of TNF-alpha and bone resorbing activity by macrophages in response to different types of bone cement particles. Biomaterials 2000;21:1005–13.
22. Wimhurst JA, Brooks RA, Rushton N. Inflammatory responses of human primary macrophages to particulate bone cements in vitro. J Bone Joint Surg Br 2001;83: 278–82.
23. Nakashima Y, Sun DH, Maloney WJ, et al. Induction of matrix metalloproteinase expression in human macrophages by orthopaedic particulate debris in vitro. J Bone Joint Surg Br 1998;80:694–700.
24. Lohmann CH, Schwartz Z, Köster G, et al. Phagocytosis of wear debris by osteoblasts affects differentiation and local factor production in a manner dependent on particle composition. Biomaterials 2000;21:551–61.
25. Vermes C, Chandrasekaran R, Jacobs JJ, et al. The effects of particulate wear debris, cytokines, and growth factors on the functions of MG-63 osteoblasts. J Bone Joint Surg Am 2001;83:201–11.
26. Lohmann CH, Dean DD, Köster G, et al. Ceramic and PMMA particles differentially affect osteoblast phenotype. Biomaterials 2002;23:1855–63.
27. Boyle WJ, Simonet WS, Lacey DL. Osteoclast differentiation and activation. Nature 2003;423(6937):337–42.
28. Goldring SR, Schiller AL, Roelke M, et al. The synovial-like membrane at the bone-cement interface in loose total hip replacements and its proposed role in bone lysis. J Bone Joint Surg Am 1983;65:575–84.
29. Haynes DR, Crotti TN, Zreiqat H. Regulation of osteoclast activity in peri-implant tissues. Biomaterials 2004;25:4877–85.
30. Udagawa N, Takahashi N, Jimi E, et al. Osteoblasts/stromal cells stimulate osteoclast activation through expression of osteoclast differentiation factor/RANKL but not macrophage colony-stimulating factor: receptor activator of NF-kappa B ligand. Bone 1999;25:517–23.
31. Haddad FS, Masri BA, Garbuz DS, et al. Femoral bone loss in total hip arthroplasty: classification and preoperative planning. Instr Course Lect 2000;49: 83–96.
32. Hodgkinson JP, Shelley P, Wroblewski BM. The correlation between the roentgenographic appearance and operative findings at the bone-cement junction of the socket in Charnley low friction arthroplasties. Clin Orthop Relat Res 1988;228: 105–9.
33. Rodrigues B, Bevernage BD, Maldague P, et al. Medium term follow-up of the AES ankle prosthesis: high rate of asymptomatic osteolysis. Foot Ankle Surg 2010;16:54–60.
34. Koivu H, Kohonen I, Sipola E, et al. Severe peri-prosthetic osteolytic lesions after the ankle evolutive system total ankle replacement. J Bone Joint Surg Br 2009;91: 907–14.
35. Koivu H, Makiewicz Z, Takakubo Y, et al. RANKL in the osteolysis of AES total ankle replacement implants. Bone 2012;51:546–52.

36. Lamberton TD, Kenny PJ, Whitehouse SL, et al. Femoral impaction grafting in revision total hip arthroplasty: a follow-up of 540 hips. J Arthroplasty 2011;26: 1154–60.
37. Halliday BR, English HW, Timmperley AJ, et al. Femoral impaction grafting with cement in revision total hip replacement. Evolution of the technique and results. J Bone Joint Surg Br 2003;85:809–17.
38. Gamradt SC, Lieberman JR. Bone graft for revision hip arthroplasty: biology and future applications. Clin Orthop Relat Res 2003;417:183–94.
39. Devries JG, Berlet GC, Lee TH, et al. Revision total ankle replacement: an early look at Agility to INBONE. Foot Ankle Spec 2011;4:235–44.
40. Myerson MS, Won HY. Primary and revision total ankle replacement using custom-designed prostheses. Foot Ankle Clin 2008;13:521–38.
41. Ketz J, Myerson MS, Sanders R. The salvage of complex hindfoot problems with use of a custom talar total ankle prosthesis. J Bone Joint Surg Am 2012;94: 1194–200.

Outcomes Following Cyst Curettage and Bone Grafting for the Management of Periprosthetic Cystic Evolution After AES Total Ankle Replacement

Jean-Luc Besse, MD, PhD[a,b,]*, Christophe Lienhart, MD[a], Michel-Henri Fessy, MD, PhD[a,b]

KEYWORDS

- Ankle arthroplasty • Bone cyst • Osteolysis • Ankle implant revision

KEY POINTS

- Bone cysts associated with total ankle replacement: Since 2008, severe medium-term cystic bone evolution was reported with AES total ankle replacement, inducing risk of mechanical complications.
- Curettage-grafting in periprosthetic cyst: The objective of the present study was to determine whether this technique provided a therapeutic solution, avoiding implant removal and arthrodesis.
- Results of the various grafts used: Iliac crest autograft, calcium phosphate cement, and polymethylmethacrylate cement were used. With a 79% functional and 92% radiological failure rate, our results in periprosthetic cyst grafting are poor. The principal surgical objective, of avoiding conversion to arthrodesis, failed in 28% of cases.
- Our present recommendations in evolutive periprosthetic cyst after total ankle replacement: We recommend annual radiological surveillance, with computed tomography (CT) in the case of increased cyst size and/or pain, so as to be able to suggest implant removal and reconstruction-arthrodesis before the talar component collapses. Onset of pain is generally related to microfracture induced by cortical lysis, detectable on CT ahead of implant migration.

[a] Department of Orthopaedic and Traumatologic Surgery, Lyon-Sud Hospital, 69 495 Pierre-Benite Cedex, France; [b] Department of Orthopedic and Traumatologic Surgery, Université Lyon 1, IFSTTAR, LBMC UMRT-9406, Centre Hospitalier Lyon-Sud, 69495 Pierre-Bénite Cédex, France
* Corresponding author. Lyon-Sud Hospital, Department of Orthopaedic and Traumatologic Surgery, 69 495 Pierre-Benite Cedex, France.
E-mail address: jean-luc.besse@chu-lyon.fr

Clin Podiatr Med Surg 30 (2013) 157–170
http://dx.doi.org/10.1016/j.cpm.2012.10.005
0891-8422/13/$ – see front matter © 2013 Elsevier Inc. All rights reserved.

podiatric.theclinics.com

INTRODUCTION

A prospective series of 50 Ankle Evolutive System (AES) total ankle replacements (TARs) (Ankle Evolutive System, Biomet, Valence, France) performed between 2003 and 2006 were evaluated in 2009 and determined to have a 29% rate of severe tibial cyst (>1 cm) and 22% talar cyst formation at 45 months of follow-up.[1] Such cystic evolution was confirmed in other series of AES TAR: Koivu and colleagues[2] reported a 21% rate of severe cyst at 31 months; Morgan and colleagues[3] reported a 24% rate of significant cyst at 58 months; Rodriguez and colleagues[4] reported a 77% rate of cyst on plain film radiographs and 100% on computed tomography (CT) imaging at 39 months; and Kokkonen and colleagues[5] reported a 79% rate of osteolysis and 40% rate of severe cyst at 28 months. Periprosthetic lysis was also reported with other 2-component[5] or 3-component TAR models.[6–9]

These cystic osteolyses induce mechanical complications due to tibial and talar cortical microfracture, notably including talar component collapse requiring reconstruction-arthrodesis.

In the present prospective series, at a minimum 6 years of follow-up, surgical revision was required in 40% of cases. We now report medium-term results for curettage-grafting in periprosthetic cyst. The objective was to determine whether this technique provided a therapeutic solution, avoiding implant removal and arthrodesis.

PATIENT SERIES

A single senior surgeon (J.L.B.) operated on a continuous prospective series of 47 patients with 50 AES TAR implants between 2003 and 2006.[1] Twenty implants involving 18 patients required revision surgery for an aspect of periprosthetic osteolysis with threatening evolution and/or onset of directly related mechanical complications.

Six implants, in 3 men and 2 women, were managed by explantation and tibiotalocalcaneal arthrodesis reconstruction: 5 for talar component fracture and subsidence and 1 because of refusal of conservative curettage-grafting.

The other revisions used conservative cyst curettage-grafting. This series comprised 14 TARs in 13 patients with a mean age of 55.6 years (range, 24–82 years) at grafting, and a predominantly male sex ratio (9:4). Indications for TAR were post-traumatic osteoarthritis in 8 cases, and osteoarthritis secondary to chronic ligament instability in 6 cases.

Mean pre-TAR American Orthopedic Foot and Ankle Surgeons Hindfoot-Ankle (AOFAS H-A) functional score[10] was 37.5 (range, 23–54). At the 1-year follow-up, functional results were satisfactory, with a mean score of 89.2 (range, 84–100); however, by the time of revision, this had fallen to a mean of 79.5. Deterioration was mainly attributable to pain; the mean score had fallen to 25.0 of 40.0 by the time of revision from 31.4 of 40.0 at 1 year after TAR. However, 43% of patients requiring revision were almost or entirely asymptomatic (pain score 30 or 40) with unchanged functional AOFAS H-A score: grafting was undertaken preventively in view of the mechanical risk posed by the size of the cysts (**Table 1**).

All patients underwent immediate postoperative anterior-posterior and lateral radiographs, repeated at 6 months and then annually. All standing radiographic views were analyzed according to the protocol of Besse and colleagues,[1] with 5 zones on the anterior-posterior view and 5 on the lateral view (**Fig. 1**). Each zone was classified as either normal, lucent (radiolucent line <2 mm), or "ballooning" osteolysis, subdivided into 5 categories according to size, with the 30-mm tibial stem as measurement reference: cyst A (osteolysis 3 to 5 mm), cyst B (osteolysis >5 mm to 1 cm), cyst C

Table 1
Series

No.	Gender	Age at Index TAR	Etiology	Preoperative AOFAS H-A (100 Points)	AOFAS H-A at 1 y	AOFAS H-A Pain (40 Points) at 1 y	Pre-graft AOFAS H-A (100 Points)	AOFAS H-A Pregraft Pain (40 Points)	Graft Date	TAR-graft Interval, mo	Etiology	Graft Type
25	M	73	Ligament instability	23	90	30	71	20	May 2008	42	Cysts	Autograft
18	M	71	Posttraumatic	40	90	30	80	20	Nov 2008	52	Cysts and cortical lysis	Autograft
11	M	21	Ligament instability	41	87	30	87	30	Dec 2008	60	Cysts	Autograft
37	F	63	Posttraumatic	54	84	30	84	30	Jan 2009	39	Cysts	Autograft
13	F	48	Posttraumatic	38	84	30	69	20	Feb 2009	60	Cysts and cortical lysis	Autograft
16	M	71	Ligament instability	45	87	30	77	20	Mar 2009	60	Cysts	Autograft
32	F	50	Ligament instability	32	87	30	74	20	Mar 2009	48	Cysts and cortical lysis	Autograft
29	M	72	Posttraumatic	40	90	30	80	20	Apr 2009	50	Cysts and cortical lysis	Autograft and PCa^{2+}
35	F	58	Ligament instability	34	90	30	90	30	Sept 2009	49	Cysts	PCa^{2+}
40	M	41	Posttraumatic	46	85	30	85	30	Oct 2009	45	Cysts and cortical lysis	PCa^{2+}
30	M	62	Posttraumatic	35	100	40	88	30	Oct 2009	57	Cysts and cortical lysis	PCa^{2+}
42	M	54	Posttraumatic	35	88	30	78	20	Apr 2010	51	Cysts	PCa^{2+}
10	M	74	Ligament instability	33	100	40	100	40	Oct 2010	70	Cysts and cortical lysis	PMMA
14	M	43	Posttraumatic	30	87	30	50	20	Oct 2011	92	Cysts and cortical lysis	PMMA

Abbreviations: AOFAS H-A, American Orthopedic Foot and Ankle Surgeons Hindfoot and Ankle Scale; No., patient number; PMMA, polymethylmethacrylate antibiotic impregnated cement; PCa^{2+}, Calcium phosphate cement.

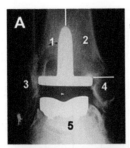
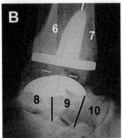

AP ankle view
- 1 : lateral Tibia
- 2 : medial Tibia
- 3 : fibular Malleolus
- 4 : medial Malleolus
- 5 : under the talar implant

Lateral ankle view
- 6 : posterior Tibial
- 7 : anterior Tibial
- 8 : post. part under the talar implant
- 9 : ant. part under the talar implant
- 10 : neck and head of Talus

Fig. 1. Radiographs showing the zones used for determining the presence and location of ballooning lysis and lucency in relation to the tibial and talar components. On anterior-posterior ankle view (A) there are 5 zones: zone 1: lateral tibia; zone 2: medial tibia; zone 3: fibular malleolus; zone 4: medial malleolus; zone 5: area under the talar implant. On lateral ankle view (B) there are 5 zones (numbers 6 through 10): zone 6: posterior tibial; zone 7: anterior tibial; zone 8: posterior area under the talar implant; zone 9: anterior area under the talar implant; zone 10: neck and head of talus.

(osteolysis >1 cm to 2 cm), cyst D (osteolysis >2 to 3 cm), or cyst E (osteolysis >3 cm). CT imaging, systematically performed ahead of TAR, at year 3 and, if necessary, ahead of revision, located, counted, and measured cysts and explored for cortical osteolysis. Eight (57%) of 14 revision cases involved cysts with cortical osteolysis on CT imaging, considered as threatening implant fracture and collapse; the other 6 had cysts with a radius larger than 3 cm, classified as severe. All showed both tibial and talar cysts.

CYST GRAFT

Mean TAR-to-revision interval was 55.3 months (range, 35–92 months). Revision used the previous anterior approach. Mean surgery time was 96 minutes (range, 65–105 minutes). Curettage was performed under visual control with a mini-image intensifier **(Fig. 2)**, guided by 3-dimensional cyst assessment on preoperative helical CT.[11] Cysts were accessed via the cortical osteolysis, when present; otherwise, a cortical bone window was performed under CT guidance. Curettage-grafting was both tibial and talar in all cases, because of systematic cyst location at both sites.

The curettage specimen was sent for histopathologic analysis, which in all cases found resorptive inflammatory foreign-body reaction infiltrate, with 94% polyethylene, 53% metallic, and 30% undetermined particles.

Spaces were then filled by compression graft. A bivalve plaster cast was fitted at postoperative day 2, for 3 weeks under non–weight bearing, followed by removable boot cast for 3 weeks, with resumption of weight bearing and physical therapy.

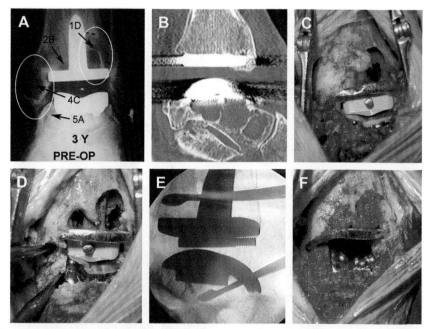

Fig. 2. Example of preventive bone graft with exchange of mobile bearing to preserve well-fixed implants (case number 25). Radiograph (*A*) and CT (*B*) assessment at 3 years for a 77-year-old man: expansile lyses and functional degradation (AOFAS H-A global score 71 vs 80 at 2 years; AOFAS H-A pain score 20 vs 30 at 2 years). Intraoperative photograph demonstrating yellow fibrous tissue in cysts (*C*). After tibial granuloma removal, implants were noted to be well fixed (*D*). Intraoperative image intensification lateral view to check talar granuloma removal (*E*). Perioperative aspect after cancellous bone autograft (*F*).

The first 7 of the 14 curettage-grafts used corticocancellous autograft from the ipsilateral anterior iliac crest, plus 1 mixed corticocancellous–calcium phosphate cement; 4 more recent procedures used calcium phosphate cement (**Fig. 3**), and the 2 most recent used polymethylmethacrylate cement (**Fig. 4**). This changeover was made in light of cyst recurrence seen on follow-up radiographs in the first autograft patients.

REVISION PROCEDURES

The functional impact of revision surgery was assessed by AOFAS H-A score[10] at the end of follow-up versus before revision: pain scores (of a maximum 40 points) were analyzed separately. Follow-up radiology comprised weight-bearing anterior-posterior and lateral views at 6 months, then annually, and CT imaging at 1 year and 3 years. Failure criteria were secondary revision, cyst recurrence, or functional deterioration.

RESULTS
Functional

There was no loss to follow-up in this prospective series. Follow-up exceeded 12 months for all but the last patient (case 14: polymethylmethacrylate cement; 9 months of follow-up), for a mean of 32 months (range, 9–47-months). Results are presented in **Table 2**.

There were no perioperative complications. One patient (number 42) showed superficial sepsis secondary to large hematoma; arthrotomy/lavage at day 20 identified no

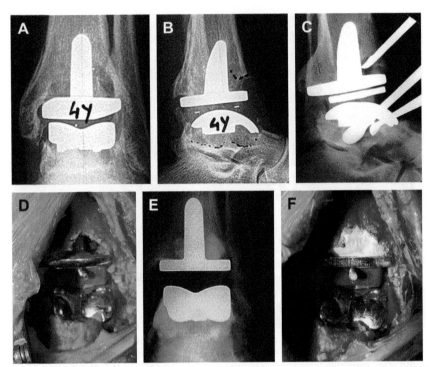

Fig. 3. Expansile cysts on anterior-posterior (*A*) and lateral (*B*) radiographs at 3 years for a 57-year-old man (case number 42). Intraoperative image intensification lateral view to check talar and tibial granuloma removal (*C*). Perioperative aspect after cyst curettage (*D*). Intraoperative image intensification assessment of calcium phosphate cement graft (*E*). Perioperative aspect of tibial and talar graft (*F*).

bacteria, but antibiotic was nevertheless instituted for 3 weeks. One case of delayed healing (number 11) resolved at 45 days with local wound care treatment.

Mean postgraft AOFAS H-A score was 65.5 (range, 21–91) and mean pain score was 17.8 (range, 0–40). In 21% of cases (numbers 10, 25, and 29), this represented an improvement in AOFAS H-A score; all patients were in pain before revision. Four patients (numbers 11, 13, 18, and 35) underwent tibiotalocalcaneal reconstruction arthrodesis (mean AOFAS H-A score, 33; pain score, 0); a fifth patient was at the time of writing considering proposed arthrodesis. If these 4 reoperated patients are excluded, mean AOFAS H-A score was 78.4 and pain score was 25, which are essentially identical to before grafting. Eleven patients (79%) showed functional failure (unimproved or worsened).

Radiological

In the 7 cases of curettage-graft by corticocancellous autograft (follow-up ≥3 years), the radiological aspect at 1 year was satisfactory, but cysts subsequently reemerged in both the talus and tibia. Three underwent arthrodesis: number18 for talar component collapse (**Fig. 5**), number 11 for progressive talar component migration into cysts larger than 30 mm, and number 13 for loosening of the tibial component and talar cyst pain. Despite their threatening cysts, 2 of these cases (numbers 10 and 25) showed good functional results and 1 (number 37) showed a moderately good result; another

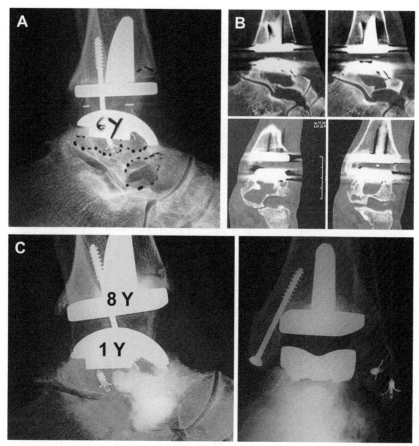

Fig. 4. Lateral radiograph (*A*) and CT assessment (*B*) at 6 years for an 81-year-old man (case number 10) demonstrating expansile talar cysts with high risk of talar subsidence, but pain free (AOFAS H-A score of 100). (*C*) Lateral and anterior-posterior radiographs at 1 year demonstrating a good radiographic result.

patient (number 16), who had a poor functional result, was at the time of writing considering proposed arthrodesis.

A single patient (number 29) had a mixed corticocancellous-calcium phosphate graft because of the severity of the bone lysis and lack of bone capital; the functional result was good, although cysts recurred in the talus.

Follow-up in the 4 calcium phosphate cement grafts exceeded 2 years. One patient (number 35) had acute infection at 12 months associated with valgus collapse attributable to medial collateral ligament failure. She underwent a 2-step revision: implant removal with antibiotic-loaded polymethylmethacrylate cement spacer and parenteral antibiotic therapy, followed 2 months later by tibiotalocalcaneal reconstruction arthrodesis (**Fig. 6**). In the other 3 (numbers 30, 40, and 42), bone-cement contact was satisfactory postoperatively, but at 1 year, a 3-mm to 5-mm lucent line emerged (**Fig. 7**), indicating nonintegration and mechanical failure; functional results were moderate in 2 of these cases and good in 1.

In the 2 patients with "salvage" cementing (number 10, who was 82 years old at revision, and number 14, who had a revision implant and showed large foreign-body

Table 2
Clinical and radiological results in whole series, according to graft type

No.	Prerevision AOFAS H-A (100 Points)	Prerevision AOFAS H-A Pain (40 Points)	Graft Type	Complications	Follow-up, mo	Radiological Result	Postrevision AOFAS H-A (100 Points)	Postrevision AOFAS H-A Pain Follow-up (40 Points)	Overall Result
25	71	20	Autograft		46	Talar cysts: 10 and 15 mm	91	40	Good but cysts
18	80	20	Autograft	Talar subsidence	41 (arthrodesis at 29)	Talar subsidence	21	0	Arthrodesis
11	87	30	Autograft		47 (arthrodesis at 47)	Tibial and talar cysts: 30 mm	32	0	Arthrodesis
37	84	30	Autograft		36	Tibial cysts	74	20	Medium
13	69	20	Autograft		46 (arthrodesis at 46)	Talar cysts and tibial lucency	43	0	Arthrodesis
16	77	20	Autograft		36	Tibial cysts: 12 and 14 mm	49	0	Suggested arthrodesis
32	74	20	Autograft		36	Tibial cysts: 17 mm	84	30	Good but cysts
29	80	20	Autograft and PCa^{2+}		36	Talar cysts: 12 mm	90	30	Good but cysts

35	90	30	PCa^{2+}	Chronic sepsis	29 (arthrodesis at 14)	Bone-cement lucency; valgus displacement	37	0	Arthrodesis
40	85	30	PCa^{2+}		25	3–5 mm bone-cement lucency	72	20	Medium
30	88	30	PCa^{2+}		24	4–5 mm bone-cement lucency; talar cysts	85	30	Good
42	78	20	PCa^{2+}	Arthrotomy lavage	24	3–5 mm bone-cement lucency	71	20	Good
10	100	40	PMMA		13	Homogeneous cement	84	30	Good
14	50	20	PMMA		9	Homogeneous cement	84	30	Good

Abbreviations: AOFAS H-A, American Orthopedic Foot and Ankle Surgeons Hindfoot and Ankle Scale; No., patient number; PMMA, polymethylmethacrylate antibiotic impregnated cement; PCa^{2+}, Calcium phosphate cement.

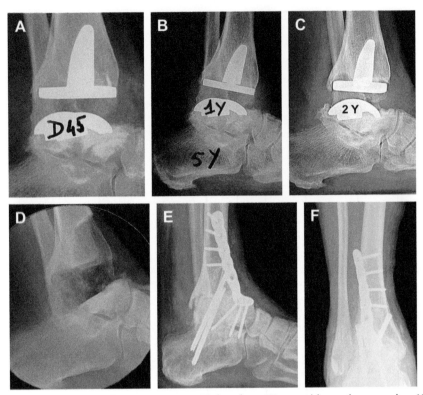

Fig. 5. Lateral radiographic assessment at 45 days for a 75-year-old man (case number 18): good radiological aspect of autograft. (*A*) A good radiological result is appreciated at 1 year, but recurrence of cyst formation in the tibia with talar component subsidence has occurred at 2 years (*B*). (*C*) Intraoperative image intensification assessment of bone defect after TAR removal and complete cyst curettage. (*D*) Note the massive osseous defect. Secondary tibiotalocalcaneal reconstruction arthrodesis with iliac crest autograft and ipsilateral intramedullary femoral corticocancellous bone autograft (using reamer-irrigator-aspirator) demonstrated on lateral (*E*) and anterior-posterior (*F*) radiographs.

granulomas exteriorized in the posterior-lateral tendon sheaths), functional results were satisfactory, although follow-up (at 9 and 13 months, respectively) was too short to foresee subsequent radiological evolution.

With 4 secondary arthrodeses, 5 cases of evolutive cyst recurrence (including 1 awaiting revision), and 3 with larger than 3-mm bone-cement radiolucency, the radiological failure rate in the present series was 92% (not counting the most recent case, number 14).

DISCUSSION

Onset of evolutive cysts complicated by fracture and implant migration results in semi-emergency arthrodesis, and led us to perform preventive surgery to halt the evolutive process and prevent mechanical dislocation, while at the same time reducing pain.[11] Functional results have been disappointing, with an improvement rate of only 21%. Radiologically, conservative management by curettage-grafting (autologous and/or calcium phosphate cement) failed to resolve the problem: 92% of the present series experienced recurrence of cyst, despite a satisfactory short-term aspect in autograft;

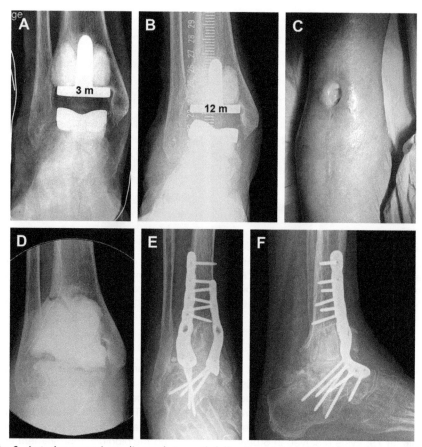

Fig. 6. Anterior-posterior radiograph 1 month following calcium phosphate cement grafting demonstrating good bone-cement contact (case number 35) (*A*). Anterior-posterior radiograph (*B*) and photograph (*C*) at 1 year demonstrating secondary valgus collapse attributable to medial collateral ligament failure associated with acute infection and granuloma recurrence. Anterior-posterior radiograph demonstrating 2-step revision: implant removal with antibiotic cement spacer (*D*) and 2 months later by tibiotalocalcaneal reconstruction arthrodesis with iliac crest autograft and ipsilateral intramedullary femoral corticocancellous bone autograft (using reamer-irrigator-aspirator) demonstrated on anterior-posterior (*E*) and lateral (*F*) radiographs.

4 cases required arthrodesis at a mean of 34 months after grafting: 2 of these were for talar component collapse, which may well threaten in the other cases of recurrence.

The strong point of the present study lies in its continuous prospective series treated by a single surgeon. All patients had regular radiographic and CT imaging follow-up studies, as recommended in the literature.[4,12] The weak points lie in the small sample size and variety of graft types. Functional results in patients without arthrodesis was unpredictable and unrelated to graft type: 3 cases improved, 3 were unchanged, and 4 worsened. Autograft and calcium phosphate cement gave comparable functional but radiographically poor results. Only the 2 patients who were managed using polymethylmethacrylate cement seemed to show good functional and satisfactory radiological results, but with insufficient follow-up for any conclusion to be drawn.

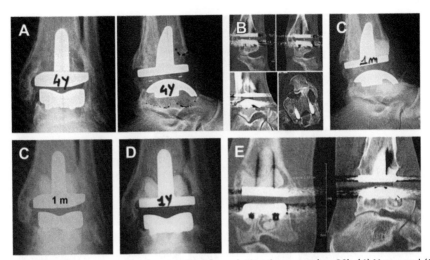

Fig. 7. Calcium phosphate (PCa) cement graft evolution (case number 30). (*A*) X-ray and (*B*) CT assessment at 4 yrs for a 57-year-old man: expansile cysts and functional degradation. (*C*) Lateral and AnteroPosterior X-ray aspect of PCa cement graft at 1 month: good bone-cement contact. 2–5 mm lucent line between PCa cement and bone on X-ray (*D*) and CT (*E*) assessment at 1 year.

Data in the literature are scarce. In 2011, at the French Society of Orthopedic Surgery and Traumatology Congress (Société Française de Chirurgie Orthopédique et Traumatologique), Trincat and Judet[13] reported a series of 322 Salto TARs, with 21 cases of painful evolutive cyst, treated by autograft. Their results at more than 2 years of follow-up differ from those in the present series: AOFAS H-A score was stable, at 79; cysts resolved in 6 patients; 11 showed radiological improvement and cyst size increased in 2 (1 of whom underwent a second graft); 2 ankles underwent arthrodesis, indicating a 19% failure rate (4/21). The discrepancy may be because of differences in TAR implant between their study and ours, and to the larger sizes of cysts in the present series. In neither series, however, did grafting improve AOFAS H-A scores over prerevision levels.

The cause of these cysts remains unclear. Stem-fixation of the tibial component has been incriminated; however, cysts also form in the talus. Implant design would not seem to be relevant, because the AES TAR (Transystem, Nimes, France and distributed by Biomet, Valence, France) and Buechel-Pappas TAR (Endotec, Orange, NJ, and Wright-Cremascoli Orthopedics [a division of Wright Medical Technologies, Europe]) models are similar in this regard, whereas the designer, Buechel and colleagues, reported 92% implant survival at 10 years[14] and Doets and colleagues (nondesigner) reported 84% implant survival at 8 years for the same model.[15]

Ultra High Molecular Weight Polyethylene can hardly be implicated in these granulomas, as it is in hip implant wear, given the early osteolytic lesions and rapid evolution without perioperative observation of any corresponding macroscopic wear of the mobile bearing.

Bonin and colleagues[8,16] suggested that some of these cysts could have evolved from osteoarthritic cysts in preexisting TAR. Curettage specimen histopathological analysis failed to confirm this hypothesis, detecting titanium and hydroxyapatite particles, in agreement with Koivu and colleagues.[2] Moreover, Bonin and colleagues[16] performed no pre-TAR CT cyst exploration, unlike in the present series, in which any cystlike formations on pre-TAR CT were discounted from analysis.[1]

The present working hypothesis was of defective primary AES implant fixation delaminating the bilayer coating, with consequent foreign-body reaction to titanium and hydroxyapatite particles, as described by Koivu and colleagues.[2] That is why foreign-body granuloma curettage was performed, taking implant integration for granted.

The main procedural risk was of implant destabilization, which would be an indication for primary arthrodesis, but which was not observed in any of the present series. It was difficult to perform curettage and complete filling of all of the cysts encountered, so as to achieve high-quality grafting: cysts were sometimes hard to access; perioperative visual control of curettage improved this step of surgery, but still could not guarantee systematic curettage of all cysts.

Apart from sometimes insufficient volume, the main problem entailed by autograft harvesting from the anterior iliac crest is the reduction in bone volume available for subsequent implant removal managed by reconstruction-arthrodesis. The calcium phosphate cement filling option proved disappointing, because of rapid onset of evolutive lucency associated with graft retraction, creating a bell-shaped aspect found in all cases in the present series. Using polymethylmethacrylate cement may seem illogical with a hydroxyapatite-coated implant, but may provide a salvage solution for elderly or multioperated patients, although follow-up at the time of writing was too short for any definitive conclusion to be drawn.

Recurrence of evolutive cyst could be caused by incomplete curettage and persistence rather than recurrence as such, given the difficulties of access, notably in the talus, and the impossibility of checking curettage quality perioperatively. It could also be caused by a continued tumorlike foreign-body effect of incrusted microparticles of titanium.

SUMMARY

With a 79% functional and 92% radiological failure rate, the present results in periprosthetic cyst grafting are poor. The principal surgical objective, of avoiding arthrodesis, failed in 28% of cases. We therefore no longer recommend this conservative preventive procedure for large and painful cysts, but rather annual radiological surveillance, with CT imaging in case of increased cyst size and/or pain, so as to be able to suggest implant removal and reconstruction-arthrodesis before the talar component collapses. Onset of pain is generally related to microfracture induced by cortical lysis, detectable on CT imaging and preceding implant migration.

REFERENCES

1. Besse JL, Brito N, Lienhart C. Clinical evaluation and radiographic assessment of bone lysis of the AES total ankle replacement. Foot Ankle Int 2009;30:964–75.
2. Koivu H, Kohonen I, Sipola E, et al. Severe periprosthetic osteolytic lesions after the ankle evolutive system total ankle replacement. J Bone Joint Surg Br 2009;91:907–14.
3. Morgan SS, Brooke B, Harris NJ. Total ankle replacement by the Ankle Evolution System: medium-term outcome. J Bone Joint Surg Br 2010;92:61–5.
4. Rodriguez D, Bevernage BD, Maldague P, et al. Medium term follow-up of the AES ankle prosthesis: high rate of asymptomatic osteolysis. Foot Ankle Surg 2010;16:54–60.

5. Kokkonen A, Ikävalko M, Tiihonen R, et al. High rate of osteolytic lesions in medium-term follow-up after the AES total ankle replacement. Foot Ankle Int 2011;32:168–75.
6. Knecht SI, Estin M, Callaghan JJ, et al. The Agility total ankle arthroplasty: seven to sixteen-year follow-up. J Bone Joint Surg Am 2004;86:1161–71.
7. Schutte BG, Louwerens JW. Short-term results of our first Scandinavian total ankle replacements (STAR). Foot Ankle Int 2008;29:124–7.
8. Bonnin M, Gaudot F, Laurent JR, et al. The Salto total ankle arthroplasty: survivorship and analysis of failures at 7 to 11 years. Clin Orthop Relat Res 2011;469:225–36.
9. Preyssas P, Toullec E, Henry M, et al. Total ankle arthroplasty: three-component total ankle arthroplasty in western France: a radiographic study. Orthop Traumatol Surg Res 2012;98(Suppl 4):S31–40.
10. Kitaoka HB, Alexander IJ, Adelaar RS, et al. Clinical rating systems for the ankle hindfoot, midfoot, hallux, and lesser toes. Foot Ankle Int 1994;15:349–53.
11. Tulberg BN, Della Valle AG. What are the guidelines for the surgical and nonsurgical treatment of periprosthetic osteolysis? J Am Acad Orthop Surg 2008;16(Suppl 1):S20–5.
12. Hanna RS, Haddad SL, Lazarus ML. Evaluation of peri-prosthetic lucency after total ankle arthroplasty: helical CT versus conventional radiography. Foot Ankle Int 2007;28:921–6.
13. Trincat S, Gaudot F, Lavigne F, et al. Prothèses totales de cheville et géodes: résultats d'autogreffes osseuses à plus de 2 ans [Total ankle arthroplasty and bone defects: results of autologous bone grafts at more than two-years]. Rev Chir Orthop Trauma 2011;97(Suppl no.7):S238–9 [in French].
14. Buechel FF Sr, Buechel FF Jr, Pappas MJ. Twenty-year evaluation of cementless mobile-bearing total ankle replacements. Clin Orthop Relat Res 2004;424:19–26.
15. Doets C, Brand R, Nelissen R. Total ankle arthroplasty in inflammatory joint disease with use of two mobile-bearing designs. J Bone Joint Surg Am 2006;88:1272–84.
16. Bonnin M, Judet T, Colombier JA, et al. Midterm results of the Salto total ankle prosthesis. Clin Orthop 2004;424:6–18.

Revision of the Aseptic and Septic Total Ankle Replacement

Norman Espinosa, MD*, Stephan Hermann Wirth, MD

KEYWORDS

- Revision • Total • Ankle • Replacement

KEY POINTS

- Total ankle replacement has become popular in the treatment of ankle osteoarthritis.
- Longevity of total ankle replacement is still limited.
- Revision total ankle replacement represents an appealing solution to maintain function and to protect the adjacent joint.
- In nonsalvageable total ankle replacement, arthrodesis is a good solution.

INTRODUCTION

In 1970, Lord and Marotte[1] were the first to implant an unconstrained cemented artificial ankle joint, which sparked interest in ankle replacements and was followed by other surgeons using a multitude of implants. As a result of an overly constrained design in combination with cemented fixation, high shear stresses along the bone-cement-implant surfaces were induced. The high shear stress led to impaired osseous integration and premature failure of total ankle replacement. As a consequence of the very high failure rate of total ankle replacement in the 1970s and 1980s, there was a period in which total ankle replacement was almost completely abandoned in clinical practice.[2,3]

A more profound understanding of ankle biomechanics and an improved design of total ankle replacements has led to the evolution of better second-generation and third-generation prostheses and resurgence of interest in this procedure. Increasing experience and availability of modern total ankle replacement has led to the stretching of indications (ie, total ankle replacement implanted in younger patients or severe deformity), which will result in a higher rate of failure than can be expected from the reported literature. Longevity of total ankle replacement remains a problem. There are few total ankle replacement designs that offer the possibility to exchange the

Department of Orthopaedic Surgery, University of Zurich, Balgrist Hospital, Forchstrasse 340, Zurich 8008, Switzerland
* Corresponding author.
E-mail address: norman.espinosa@balgrist.ch

Clin Podiatr Med Surg 30 (2013) 171–185
http://dx.doi.org/10.1016/j.cpm.2012.10.004
0891-8422/13/$ – see front matter © 2013 Elsevier Inc. All rights reserved.

prosthesis, and few surgeons have experience with revision total ankle replacement. Therefore, in the case of a failed total ankle replacement, conversion to an ankle arthrodesis has remained the gold standard. However, arthrodesis of the ankle joint leads to abnormal biomechanical transmissions of forces and gait alterations. As a result, the adjacent joints compensate for the loss of motion and become overloaded and arthritic, and therefore the use of ankle fusion should be weighted critically.[4] In order to preserve motion at the ankle, and thus to protect the adjacent subtalar and mid-tarsal joints, the ability to exchange the implant successfully is desirable. However, there is sparse information in the literature regarding revision total ankle replacement.[5,6]

BIOMECHANICAL ASPECTS OF TOTAL ANKLE REPLACEMENT BEHAVIOR AND FAILURE

During normal gait the ankle joint is loaded with a force approximately 6 times body weight.[7] This force is reduced to 3 times body weight in a degenerated ankle joint.[8] However, it is assumed that for total ankle replacement, the strength of bone should be at least 3 times greater than in normal conditions. Proper fixation techniques are needed to compensate for those forces exerted under high-performance activities to avoid any subsidence of the components. In addition, under optimal conditions, the ultrahigh-molecular-weight polyethylene (UHMWPE) insert should be as thick as possible to avoid premature wear. UHMWPE wear depends on geometry, strength (ultrastructure), and alignment of the components.[9] At present, there is no appropriate recommendation about the UHMWPE thickness that should be used in total ankle replacement. From a logical standpoint, an optimal UHMWPE insert should be thin and strong without the risk of impairing bony strength at the bone-implant interface. In addition, a perfect prosthesis should replicate the ankle joint in an anatomic way and mimic kinetics and kinematics of a normal joint.[10–12] Thus, a total ankle replacement should maximize conformity and optimize constraint. The high conformity of bearing surfaces avoids peak pressures and wear. In contrast, an artificial ankle joint needs sufficient constraint to provide stability but without increasing shear stresses at the bone-implant interface, which could lead to premature failure of the implant. Contemporary 3-component total ankle replacement designs are more anatomic, present improved biomechanical performance, and use biologic integration of the components.[13,14] The surfaces are covered with calcium-hydroxyapatite variably combined with the porous coating of the component. The advantages of an anatomic design and biologic cementless fixation include less extensive resections of the tibia and talus, smaller sizes of implants, reduction of body wear, and avoidance of heat destruction of the soft tissues and bones. These advantages make revision total ankle replacement and easier conversion into an ankle arthrodesis after failed primary total ankle replacement a possibility. Although the results of cemented and uncemented first-generation total ankle replacement designs were limited and disappointing, contemporary third-generation 3-component designs with meniscal bearing fulfill anatomic and biomechanically sound criteria. A more anatomically designed total ankle replacement better replicates the normal ankle joint range of motion with better tolerance of congruent mobile bearing designs with regard to malalignment and even pressure distribution within the ankle joint compared with a 2-component fixed bearing design.[10–12,15]

When a total ankle replacement becomes loose, the tibial and talar components behave abnormally with increased motion in the frontal, transverse, and sagittal planes. This abnormal movement of components results in increased stress transmission across the supporting bone. According to Wolff's law, remodeling processes take place resulting in either strengthening or weakening of the osseous ultrastructure.

In the case of tibial component loosening, the ring-shaped cortex at the metaphysis of the tibia becomes sclerotic and, in the center, a reduction of cancellous bone mass or formation of cysts takes place. Some total ankle replacement designs include fixation stems (eg, STAR Ankle, Small Bone Innovations, Inc, Morrisville, PA; INBONE, Wright Medical Technology, Arlington, TN; Mobility, DePuy Orthopedics, Warsaw, IN; Salto Tolaris, Tornier, Edina, MN). It is important to anticipate greater bone defects in these types of total ankle replacement during removal of the implant.[16] Therefore, a flat revision component of the tibia that holds well against the cortical ring of the tibial metaphysis and does not rely on the weakened or absent cancellous bone is preferred. This cortical rim support provides enough support to act against possible tibial subsidence. In the case of talar component loosening, the component starts to swing in an anterior-posterior and proximal-distal fashion. This effect results in condensed or sclerotic bone mass in the anterior and posterior parts of the talus. These locations are also where cyst formations can be found.

REVISION RATES OF CONTEMPORARY TOTAL ANKLE REPLACEMENT DESIGNS

The design of a total ankle replacement plays an important role in its biomechanical behavior and therefore influences overall results.[3] Recently published short-term and midterm data for the HINTEGRA (NEWDEAL International, Lyon, France), a highly anatomic design, showed revision rates of approximately 7% to 14%.[13,17] These rates are less than the 23% revision rate identified by SooHoo and colleagues.[18] More sophisticated techniques and improved instrumentation combined with the experience of a surgeon can achieve low infection rates (3% superficial, 1% deep). Hintermann and colleagues[17] reported loosening of the talar component in 5.5% of cases. However, almost no loosening of the tibial component was observed (0.7%). Henricson and colleagues[19,20] reported revision rates for the HINTEGRA between 14% and 22%.[19,20] In contrast, the short-term results for the first 100 Mobility total ankle replacements (DePuy Orthopedics, Inc. Warsaw, IN) were reported by Wood and colleagues[21] and the revision rate was even lower (5%) than that reported by Hintermann and colleagues.[17] However, 10-year survival rates of the HINTEGRA or Mobility total ankle replacements are currently not available. Long-term studies are needed to prove whether those designs show any superior behavior and outcome compared with the 2-component and 3-component total ankle replacement designs that are presently available. The direct comparison between HINTEGRA and Mobility total ankle replacements did not reveal any difference regarding complication rates.[14,22] Both designs preserve enough bone stock and the HINTEGRA design offers the possibility of revision total ankle replacement.[22] More recently, Schenk and colleagues[23] presented the results of 401 Salto Tolaris total ankle replacements after a mean follow-up of 29 months. The calculated 5-year survivorship was 88% and the revision rate 11%. Regarding the STAR Ankle, there are numerous reports in the literature. With specific focus on revision rate, values ranging between 14% and 48% for single-coating designs and 7% and 24% for double-coated designs have been derived from national registries in Scandinavia.[24,25] Nunley and colleagues[26] recently reported a low revision rate for the STAR Ankle, averaging 6%.

GENERAL THOUGHTS ON REVISION TOTAL ANKLE REPLACEMENT

Reasons for total ankle replacement failure include aseptic and septic loosening.[27] Aseptic loosening may occur secondary to poor osseous integration, inaccurate sizing, malalignment, and UHMWPE insert wear.[15] The surgeon performing revision surgery faces serious problems. Loss of bone stock occurs as a result of resection for prosthetic implantation and/or secondary wear with periprosthetic osteolysis. In addition, the soft tissue is vulnerable, especially in rheumatoid patients, making salvage surgery at the ankle more difficult than revision of failed total ankle replacements in other joints. In addition, variable degrees of fixed hindfoot deformities and contractures, which may be caused by concomitant subtalar osteoarthritis and tibial or talar component subsidence, can complicate revision surgery.[22] The presence of poor bone quality impairs fixation and therefore specific fixation strategies must be selected. Any imbalance at the ankle must be detected and addressed to prevent malalignment of the total ankle replacement, which has detrimental effects on longevity of the implant if not corrected.[15,22,28] This process includes assessment of possible incompetence of the lateral or medial ligaments. Osteotomies or arthrodesis are occasionally required to balance and stabilize the hindfoot to restore and maintain neutral alignment.

Therefore the most important question is whether the surgeon can implant a new total ankle replacement under stable conditions.

There is a paucity of reports in the literature regarding the treatment of failed total ankle replacement, with no clear indication of how to proceed in such difficult cases.[5,6,29] There are certain thoughts that should be considered before embarking on revision total ankle replacement. **Table 1** lists some principles, as discussed by Hintermann and colleagues.[22] As long as those thoughts are considered, revision total ankle replacement is likely to be successful. Septic loosening of total ankle replacement is a serious condition that affects not only the osseous but also the soft tissue parts. Despite this, it can lead to serious systemic and life-threatening medical conditions if not treated well. As such, the indication to revise such an ankle is more aggressive than that for an aseptic loosening.

PREOPERATIVE ASSESSMENT

The patient should be examined barefoot during walking and in a standing position, followed by evaluation of leg and hindfoot alignment. Equinus contracture involving either the gastrocnemius or the Achilles tendon should be determined because they may play an important role in correcting the hindfoot and must be addressed surgically

Table 1 Considerations for total ankle replacement revision surgery	
Osseous support	The components should be placed on well-perfused and viable bone stock A 3-point support is optimal for stability Any osseous defect should be filled with either autogenous graft or allograft
Ligamentous tensioning	The goal is to restore the joint line The larger a bone defect, the greater the components or custom-made components Medial malleolar or fibular osteotomies might be considered to improve ligament tension Ligament reconstructions can help to improve stability at the ankle
Hindfoot alignment	A correctly aligned hindfoot supports a balanced total ankle replacement Corrective osteotomies should be liberally used Fusions of the hindfoot and midfoot can be necessary to create a stable and well-aligned socket for total ankle replacement

if present. Potential deformities (eg, varus or valgus malalignment and midfoot prona-
tion or supination) and their flexibility are assessed. Rotatory alignment of the hindfoot
is assessed using both malleoli to mark out the axis and comparing it with the patella.
In addition, the condition of the soft tissues and neurovascular status must be
evaluated.

Performance of standardized weight-bearing anterior-posterior and lateral radiographs of the ankle follows the thorough clinical examination. The hindfoot alignment
views as described by Saltzman and colleagues or, preferably, a long leg axial view
are used to assess any valgus or varus deformity and to evaluate prosthetic migration
and bone loss.[30–32] In order to rule out adjacent joint arthritis and to assess possible
peritalar instability, anterior-posterior and lateral views of the foot are mandatory. The
anterior-posterior and lateral views of the ankle allow proper assessment of the tibial
component in the frontal and sagittal plane. However, the bone stock underneath the
talar component cannot be accurately determined with plain radiographs. In those
cases, computed tomography (CT) is helpful to determine the extent of bony destruction
and to anticipate possible need for grafts or custom-made total ankle replacement
components (when there is insufficient remaining talus). The use of single-photon emission CT and fluorodeoxyglucose positron emission CT might be helpful to identify pathologic processes around the total ankle replacement components.[33–35]

SURGICAL MANAGEMENT

If the joint can be preserved/salvaged, the authors also use the HINTEGRA total ankle
replacement system (Newdeal, Lyon, France) for primary and revision total ankle
replacement. When considering revision total ankle replacement, the authors refer
to an algorithm proposed by Hintermann and colleagues,[22] which is based on the
size of bony defect at either the tibial or talar site. The standard tibial component of
the HINTEGRA has a thickness of 4 mm. There are revision tibial components available
with 8-mm and 12-mm thickness but they are not frequently used because most revision cases can be addressed by sole implantation of a standard tibial component. The
talar revision component has a flat undersurface and long pegs to provide strong fixation within the talar bone. The shape of the talar component is conical with different
medial and lateral radii, and therefore is as anatomic as possible. The technique of
revision total ankle replacement using the HINTEGRA system as performed by the
senior author is described later.[36]

The same anterior approach as used in the primary total ankle replacement is used.
The skin conditions in the anterior part of the ankle joint are critical. Careful handling of
the soft tissues is mandatory to prevent wound healing problems such as skin
necrosis. Therefore, no sharp forceps or retractors are used during surgery. Any thick-
ened scar tissue in front of the total ankle replacement needs to be removed and, at
times, there is also the necessity to remove osseous debris to access the failed total
ankle replacement. To remove the total ankle replacement from the underlying bone it
is recommended to use osteotomes or chisels. In our daily practice, we always obtain
3 different samples of tissue, which are sent to pathology to rule out or to confirm an
infectious process. In cases of septic loosening and/or purulent infection, a 2-stage
procedure is performed starting with removal of the total ankle replacement and insertion of an antibiotic-loaded polymethyl methacrylate cement spacer. If it is not
possible to salvage the infected total ankle replacement, a 2-staged conversion
to an arthrodesis should be considered. Patients who qualify for ankle arthrodesis
are those with aseptic loosening of their total ankle replacement and/or eradicated
prosthetic joint infection associated with a massive bone loss and the unfeasibility

of revision total ankle replacement. In general, patients suffering from early prosthetic joint infection (ie, present for less than 3 weeks), with high susceptibility of the microorganisms against antibiotics, good soft tissue conditions, and adequate implant stability could be treated by retention of the implant. Otherwise prosthetic joint infection results in implant removal. If the implant is removed, the prosthetic components are removed and the joint debrided, followed by implantation of an antibiotic-loaded cement spacer. Adequate parenteral antibiotic treatment is administered for 4 to 8 weeks. After this period, antibiotic treatment is halted and the infectious parameters checked to make sure that infection no longer exists. In the absence of infection, ankle arthrodesis can be considered. **Fig. 1** shows an algorithm of how to approach the infected total ankle replacement.[27]

If the prosthetic implant can be retained, the total ankle replacement components are carefully removed while avoiding further damage to the adjacent osseous structures. In total ankle replacement with tibial stems, it is necessary to create anterior cortical windows. It is crucial to limit this window to a minimum because any resection of the anterior distal tibia cortex weakens the bone and therefore impairs fixation of subsequent total ankle replacement. This step is followed by a thorough inspection of the tibial and talar remnants. Cysts are debrided until the subchondral bone plate is visible. Then the cysts are filled with either allograft or autograft bone impacted into place. For this purpose, a surgeon might have to harvest bone from the proximal tibia or iliac crest. The medial and lateral gutters of the ankle are then cleaned out. The posterior capsule is resected while avoiding the neurovascular structures at the posteromedial aspect of the ankle. By means of the alignment jig of the revision total ankle replacement, the tibial cut is made from anterior to posterior. The tibial resection should be limited to a minimum. The goal is to obtain a flat cut while preserving the

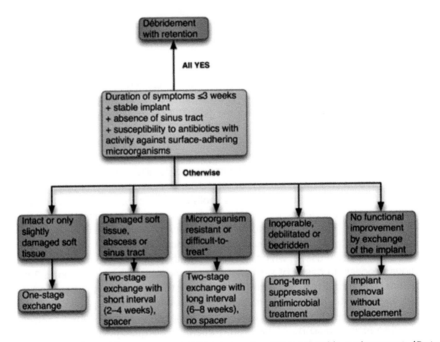

Fig. 1. An algorithm of how to proceed in a case of septic total ankle replacement. (*Data from* Refs.[16,43–46])

cortical ring of the tibial metaphysis. The talar cut is made flat and parallel to the tibial plane. Using a distractor on the medial part of the ankle joint, neutral alignment with balanced ligamentous tension is achieved. Sometimes release of the collateral ligaments is needed to achieve proper balance. The distance between the tibial and talar surfaces is measured. According to Hintermann and colleagues,[22] in the case of a distance up to 18 mm, standard tibial and talar components can be used (**Fig. 2**). When the gap is greater than 18 mm but is less than 25 mm, a standard tibial and revision component can be used. Gaps with distances more than 25 mm and almost no talar body left require custom-made revision total ankle replacement components. If the tibial cut is too large, a revision tibial component should be considered, which is fixed with 2 screws placed from anterior to posterior. The trial components are inserted and the stability of the ankle joint is checked. Once a stable condition is achieved, the final components are inserted. Sometimes it is necessary to fill the medial and lateral gutters with autologous or allogenic bone graft to enhance stability (**Fig. 3**).

ADDITIONAL SURGERY

Malalignment and other potential reasons for instability should be addressed at the time when revision total ankle replacement is performed. Adjusting the tibial cuts can compensate a varus or valgus malalignment of up to 10°. Greater deformities should be corrected either by supramalleolar (closing or open wedge) or calcaneal osteotomies (medial or lateral sliding or Z-shaped). Discrepancies in fibular length are addressed by distraction together with bone block insertion (if too short) or shortening (if too long) (**Fig. 4**). In the case of lateral ligamentous instability, a repair of the anterior talofibular ligament, the calcaneofibular ligament, or both should be

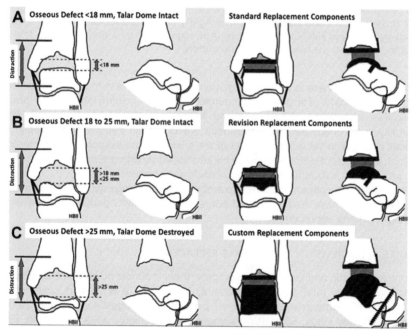

Fig. 2. Decision making in a case of loss of bone stock. (*From* Hintermann B, Barg A, Knupp M. [Revision arthroplasty of the ankle joint]. Orthopäde 2011;40(11):1000–7. [in German]; with permission.)

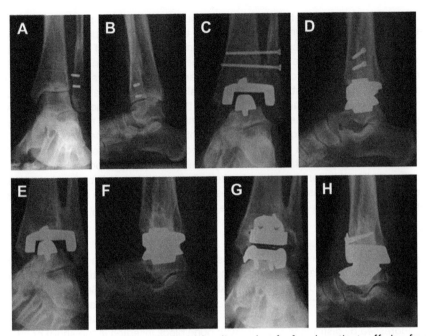

Fig. 3. Anterior-posterior (*A*) and lateral (*B*) radiographs of a female patient suffering from symptomatic posttraumatic ankle osteoarthritis following plate and screw removal. Anterior-posterior (*C*) and lateral (*D*) radiographs after implantation of an Agility total ankle replacement. Anterior-posterior (*E*) and lateral (*F*) radiographs 5 years after surgery with painful aseptic osteolysis and pain. Anterior-posterior (*G*) and lateral (*H*) radiographs after revision total ankle replacement. The Agility total ankle replacement has been replaced by a revision HINTEGRA prosthesis. Autologous iliac crest graft has been inserted to fill the defects in the medial and lateral gutters.

performed. When there is no viable ligament tissue left, reconstruction of the lateral ligaments by transfer of an allogenic or autologous free hamstring tendon graft (gracilis or semitendinosus) should be considered. In the case of marked anterolateral ankle instability, a peroneus longus to peroneus brevis tendon transfer can be effective. Arthritic changes in the adjacent joints of the ankle that are associated with hindfoot, midfoot, and forefoot deformity should be addressed by arthrodesis to create a stable and well-aligned socket for revision total ankle replacement.

After surgery, the patient is allowed to ambulate in a walking cast or removable boot. In patients who have had additional surgery on their feet, partial or non–weight-bearing regimens are recommended.

RESULTS AFTER REVISION TOTAL ANKLE REPLACEMENT

In contrast with hip and knee revision surgery, there is almost no information available regarding revision total ankle replacement; information is limited to case reports only.[5,6,29,37] Hintermann and colleagues[22] published the largest series in the German literature. In their study, 83 revision surgeries in 79 patients were performed. Fifty-three percent of cases revealed an aseptic loosening, 41% suffered from painful dysfunction, and 6% from a septic loosening of the total ankle replacement. Five-years after surgery, 83% of patients were satisfied with the result, 14% judged the

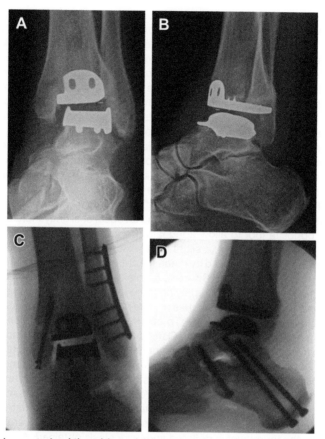

Fig. 4. Anterior-posterior (*A*) and lateral (*B*) radiographs following HINTEGRA total ankle replacement in a male patient suffering from a pes cavovarus foot deformity and unrecognized peritalar instability as shown by parallelism between the talus and the calcaneus. Note the remarkable varus malalignment. Anterior-posterior (*C*) and lateral (*D*) intraoperative image intensification views following derotational subtalar arthrodesis and revision total ankle replacement (tibial component). Note that the talus and its relationship to the tibia and calcaneus have been improved. In addition, to balance the hindfoot a fibular lengthening osteotomy with interposition of allogenic bone graft has been performed and secured with 2 screws. A shortening fibular osteotomy has been added to correct hindfoot axis. Note the correct alignment of the hindfoot.

result as fair, and 2% as poor. Of all patients, 59% were pain free at time of follow-up with an acceptable range of motion at the ankle joint (34°). In addition to exchange of the metallic components, 36 concomitant procedures (ie, arthrodesis, osteotomies, ligament repairs, and peroneus longus to peroneus brevis transfers) were performed to balance the hindfoot.

WHEN ARTHRODESIS IS REQUIRED

If a total ankle replacement cannot be retained, arthrodesis represents a viable solution. We prefer to use an anterior compression plating system.[16,27] The septic total ankle replacement is approached through an approximately 10-cm longitudinal incision, which is made over the anterior aspect of the ankle joint. Care is taken not to injure the superficial peroneal nerve and its terminal branches. The sheath of the anterior tibial tendon is opened laterally together with the proximal extensor retinaculum. The incision is deepened between the tendons of the anterior tibial and extensor hallucis longus muscles. The neurovascular bundle is retracted laterally together with the extensor hallucis longus tendon. The joint capsule and periosteum are incised. A laminar spreader is inserted medially into the tibia and talus and the total ankle replacement explored. In the case of component loosening, hardware removal can be achieved with a chisel. Areas of remaining fibrous, sclerotic, and necrotic tissue must be debrided by means of an oscillating saw (to create even surfaces) and/or curette and chisel until vital subchondral bone is available. The surfaces of the tibia, talus, and fibular are drilled with a 2-mm drill. Depending on the magnitude of bone loss, tricortical iliac crest autograft only or a combination of iliac crest autograft and femoral head allograft is used. The defect zone is bridged by means of the bone graft(s). The surfaces are compressed while carefully checking the hindfoot position. The desired alignment of an arthrodesis is neutral dorsiflexion, 5° of hindfoot valgus, and an equal or slightly more external rotation than the opposite foot to allow adequate propulsion over the medial ray at final stance. In a completely stiff foot, a slight dorsiflexion position of the ankle joint could be considered. Fixation is achieved by means of anterior double plating. Double plating can either be done by using two 3.5-mm, 5-hole to 6-hole, limited contact dynamic compression titanium plates or by applying more anatomic designs (Tibaxys System, Newdeal, Lyon, France). Both techniques use the plates, with 1 being placed anterolateral and the other more anteromedial. To obtain adequate compression, we recommend using an Arbeitsgemeinschaft fur Osteosynthesefragen (AO) tensioning device. Together with the Achilles tendon, the anterior double-plating system acts as a tension band system that puts the ankle joint under maximum but evenly distributed compression. The fibular is fixed to the tibia and talus with 2 to 3 titanium screws (3.5 mm). Cancellous bone graft is harvested from the proximal tibia or iliac crest. After thorough irrigation, the cancellous bone is circumferentially inserted, filling all defects, building a bridge of autologous bone between the distal tibia and the talar remnant. Before wound closure, the tourniquet is deflated and hemostasis obtained. A closed suction drain is inserted to prevent hematoma formation. The joint capsule and the tendon sheaths as well as the subcutaneous tissues are closed with single monofilament absorbable sutures and the skin is closed with a single nonabsorbable suture. A split short leg plaster cast is applied over a sterile dressing.

The patient is kept in bed for 48 hours with the operated leg elevated. After this time, a well-padded removable short leg cast is applied. The patient is mobilized on 2 crutches and is non–weight bearing until complete wound healing is verified. When verified, the patient can augment weight bearing up to 15 to 25 kg for an additional 6 weeks. Sutures are removed after 2 weeks. At 8 weeks after surgery, the patient is checked clinically and radiographically. If radiographic assessment shows sufficient signs of osseous consolidation at this point, weight bearing is progressively increased. Full healing might take 3 to 6 months. If there is any doubt of consolidation and bone graft integration, we recommend the performance of CT. Deep venous thrombosis prophylaxis should be continued until cast-free full weight bearing is achieved. The patient is provided with shoe modifications to improve the gait pattern and to save the adjacent joints from early overload and progressive arthrosis.

RESULTS AFTER FUSION

Little information is available regarding the management of failed total ankle replacement by means of ankle arthrodesis. Zwipp and Grass[38] reported on 4 patients undergoing ankle arthrodesis after failed total ankle replacement. Two of them were done by screw fixation alone, whereas the remaining 2 failures were treated by anterior plating using two 3.5-mm limited contact dynamic compression titanium plates. Of the latter, 1 patient needed revision surgery because of nonunion. Groth and Fitch[39] described ankle arthrodesis without bone grafting. However, such a procedure leads to significant shortening. Hopgood and colleagues[40] published their report on 23 ankles that were converted to arthrodesis. Among those there were only 8 cases that used compression screw fixation, but all of them achieved complete union. In patients with rheumatoid arthritis, tibiotalocalcaneal arthrodesis performed better than ankle fusion alone. The investigators of the same study also stated that total ankle replacement design plays an important role in determining whether larger bone grafts should be used to bridge the gap. The more resurfacing the total ankle replacement

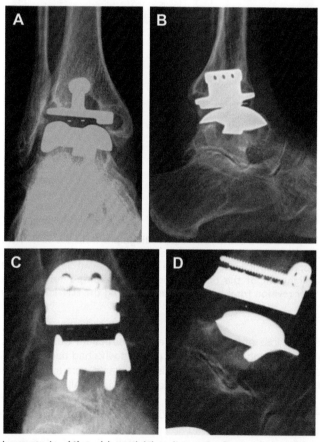

Fig. 5. Anterior-posterior (A) and lateral (B) radiographs from a hemophilic male patient who received a right Salto Tolaris total ankle replacement 6 years ago. At the time of presentation the patient suffered from pain and the radiographs reveal aseptic loosening of the components with large osteolytic reactions and malalignment of the tibial component. Anterior-posterior (C) and lateral (D) radiographs after revision total ankle replacement using the HINTEGRA system with revision components. Note the tibial revision component with a greater thickness than the standard one and the longer pegs for the talar component.

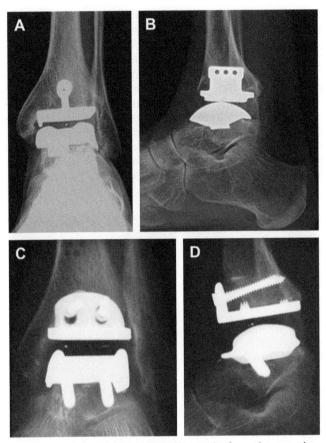

Fig. 6. Anterior-posterior (*A*) and lateral (*B*) radiographs from the same hemophilic male patient depicted in **Fig. 5** who received a left Salto Tolaris total ankle replacement that had also developed aseptic loosening of the components with less severe osteolytic reactions and malalignment of the tibial component. Anterior-posterior (*C*) and lateral (*D*) radiographs after revision total ankle replacement using the HINTEGRA system with standard components.

has, the less bone loss and the easier the reconstruction. Culpan and colleagues[41] presented a more homogenous series of patients who had had conversion of failed total ankle replacement in ankle arthrodesis. All patients were treated using compression screw fusion with use of tricortical iliac crest grafts. All patients but 1 achieved solid union and no complications were reported. More recently, Berkowitz and colleagues[42] reported on salvage arthrodesis after failed total ankle replacement. They compared 12 patients who had an ankle fusion with 12 patients who had tibiotalocalcaneal arthrodesis. In the group with tibiotalocalcaneal arthrodesis, nonunions occurred and were identified as a risk factor for worse outcome.

SUMMARY

Contemporary third-generation designs of total ankle replacement provide improved anatomic and biomechanical behavior. However, their longevity is limited and even the best total ankle replacement can fail at some point and need revision surgery.

Conversion into arthrodesis has remained the mainstay in treating failed total ankle replacement but at the cost of function of the hindfoot. In order to preserve hindfoot motion and function while protecting the adjacent joints, the idea of total ankle replacement exchange is appealing. Current total ankle replacement systems offer the possibility to revise and exchange parts or the complete implant (**Figs. 5** and **6**). It is important to perform a thorough preoperative evaluation before embarking on revision total ankle replacement. Associated disorders, such as, extra-articular malalignment, instability, and potential causes of impingement, should be identified and corrected at the same time. Recent reports including larger patient populations are encouraging. The future will show whether revision total ankle replacement will yield similar results to those seen in hip and knee surgery. When there is no chance to preserve the total ankle replacement, salvage arthrodesis remains a viable option with reasonable results.

REFERENCES

1. Lord G, Marotte JH. Total ankle prosthesis. Technique and 1st results. Apropos of 12 cases. Rev Chir Orthop Reparatrice Appar Mot 1973;59(2):139–51 [in French].
2. Jensen NC, Kroner K. Total ankle joint replacement: a clinical follow up. Orthopedics 1992;15(2):236–9.
3. Cracchiolo A 3rd, Deorio JK. Design features of current total ankle replacements: implants and instrumentation. J Am Acad Orthop Surg 2008;16(9):530–40.
4. Coester LM, Saltzman CL, Leupold J, et al. Long-term results following ankle arthrodesis for post-traumatic arthritis. J Bone Joint Surg Am 2001;83(2):219–28.
5. Kharwadkar N, Harris NJ. Revision of STAR total ankle replacement to hybrid AES-STAR total ankle replacement-a report of two cases. Foot Ankle Surg 2009;15(2):101–5.
6. Assal M, Greisberg J, Hansen ST Jr. Revision total ankle arthroplasty: conversion of New Jersey low contact stress to agility: surgical technique and case report. Foot Ankle Int 2004;25(12):922–5.
7. Perry J, Schoneberger B. Gait analysis: normal and pathological function. Edited. Thorofare (NJ): Slack Inc; 1992.
8. Valderrabano V, Nigg BM, von Tscharner V, et al. Gait analysis in ankle osteoarthritis and total ankle replacement. Clin Biomech 2007;22(8):894–904.
9. Gill LH. Principles of joint arthroplasty as applied to the ankle. Instr Course Lect 2002;51:117–28.
10. Valderrabano V, Hintermann B, Nigg BM, et al. Kinematic changes after fusion and total replacement of the ankle: part 3: talar movement. Foot Ankle Int 2003;24(12):897–900.
11. Valderrabano V, Hintermann B, Nigg BM, et al. Kinematic changes after fusion and total replacement of the ankle: part 2: movement transfer. Foot Ankle Int 2003;24(12):888–96.
12. Valderrabano V, Hintermann B, Nigg BM, et al. Kinematic changes after fusion and total replacement of the ankle: part 1: range of motion. Foot Ankle Int 2003;24(12):881–7.
13. Hintermann B, Valderrabano V, Dereymaeker G, et al. The HINTEGRA ankle: rationale and short-term results of 122 consecutive ankles. Clin Orthop Relat Res 2004;424:57–68.
14. Lee KT, Lee YK, Young KW, et al. Perioperative complications of the MOBILITY total ankle system: comparison with the HINTEGRA total ankle system. J Orthop Sci 2010;15(3):317–22.

15. Espinosa N, Walti M, Favre P, et al. Misalignment of total ankle components can induce high joint contact pressures. J Bone Joint Surg Am 2010;92(5): 1179–87.
16. Espinosa N, Wirth S, Jankauskas L. Ankle fusion after failed total ankle replacement. Tech Foot Ankle Surg 2010;9(4):199–204.
17. Hintermann B, Valderrabano V, Knupp M, et al. The HINTEGRA ankle: short- and mid-term results. Orthopade 2006;35(5):533–45 [in German].
18. SooHoo NF, Zingmond DS, Ko CY. Comparison of reoperation rates following ankle arthrodesis and total ankle arthroplasty. J Bone Joint Surg Am 2007; 89(10):2143–9.
19. Henricson A, Carlsson A, Rydholm U. What is a revision of total ankle replacement? Foot Ankle Surg 2011;17(3):99–102.
20. Henricson A, Skoog A, Carlsson A. The Swedish ankle arthroplasty register: an analysis of 531 arthroplasties between 1993 and 2005. Acta Orthop 2007; 78(5):569–74.
21. Wood PL, Karski MT, Watmough P. Total ankle replacement: the results of 100 mobility total ankle replacements. J Bone Joint Surg Br 2010;92(7):958–62.
22. Hintermann B, Barg A, Knupp M. Revision arthroplasty of the ankle joint. Orthopade 2011;40(11):1000–7 [in German].
23. Schenk K, Lieske S, John M, et al. Prospective study of a cementless, mobile-bearing, third generation total ankle prosthesis. Foot Ankle Int 2011;32(8):755–63.
24. Fevang BT, Lie SA, Havelin LI, et al. 257 ankle arthroplasties performed in Norway between 1994 and 2005. Acta Orthop 2007;78(5):575–83.
25. Skytta ET, Koivu H, Eskelinen A, et al. Total ankle replacement: a population-based study of 515 cases from the Finnish Arthroplasty Register. Acta Orthop 2010;81(1):114–8.
26. Nunley JA, Caputo AM, Easley ME, et al. Intermediate to long-term outcomes of the STAR total ankle replacement: the patient perspective. J Bone Joint Surg Am 2012;94(1):43–8.
27. Espinosa N, Wirth SH. Ankle arthrodesis after failed total ankle replacement. Orthopade 2011;40(11):1008–17 [in German].
28. Klammer G, Benninger E, Espinosa N. The varus ankle and instability. Foot Ankle Clin 2012;17(1):57–82.
29. Myerson MS, Won HY. Primary and revision total ankle replacement using custom-designed prostheses. Foot Ankle Clin 2008;13(3):521–38.
30. Buck FM, Hoffmann A, Mamisch-Saupe N, et al. Hindfoot alignment measurements: rotation-stability of measurement techniques on hindfoot alignment view and long axial view radiographs. AJR Am J Roentgenol 2011;197(3):578–82.
31. Reilingh ML, Beimers L, Tuijthof GJ, et al. Measuring hindfoot alignment radiographically: the long axial view is more reliable than the hindfoot alignment view. Skeletal Radiol 2010;39(11):1103–8.
32. Saltzman CL, el-Khoury GY. The hindfoot alignment view. Foot Ankle Int 1995; 16(9):572–6.
33. Knupp M, Pagenstert GI, Barg A, et al. SPECT-CT compared with conventional imaging modalities for the assessment of the varus and valgus malaligned hindfoot. J Orthop Res 2009;27(11):1461–6.
34. Pagenstert GI, Barg A, Leumann AG, et al. SPECT-CT imaging in degenerative joint disease of the foot and ankle. J Bone Joint Surg Br 2009;91(9):1191–6.
35. Fischer DR, Maquieira GJ, Espinosa N, et al. Therapeutic impact of [(18)F]fluoride positron-emission tomography/computed tomography on patients with unclear foot pain. Skeletal Radiol 2010;39(10):987–97.

36. Hintermann B. Total ankle arthroplasty: historical overview, current concepts and future perspectives. Edited. Vienna (NY): Springer-Verlag; 2005.
37. Gould JS. Revision total ankle arthroplasty. Am J Orthop 2005;34(8):361.
38. Zwipp H, Grass R. Ankle arthrodesis after failed joint replacement. Oper Orthop Traumatol 2005;17(4–5):518–33 [in English, German].
39. Groth HE, Fitch HF. Salvage procedures for complications of total ankle arthroplasty. Clin Orthop Relat Res 1987;224:244–50.
40. Hopgood P, Kumar R, Wood PL. Ankle arthrodesis for failed total ankle replacement. J Bone Joint Surg Br 2006;88(8):1032–8.
41. Culpan P, Le Strat V, Piriou P, et al. Arthrodesis after failed total ankle replacement. J Bone Joint Surg Br 2007;89(9):1178–83.
42. Berkowitz MJ, Clare MP, Walling AK, et al. Salvage of failed total ankle arthroplasty with fusion using structural allograft and internal fixation. Foot Ankle Int 2011;32(5):493–502.
43. Trampuz A, Zimmerli W. Prosthetic joint infections: update in diagnosis and treatment. Swiss Med Wkly 2005;135(17–18):243–51.
44. Trampuz A, Zimmerli W. New strategies for the treatment of infections associated with prosthetic joints. Curr Opin Investig Drugs 2005;6(2):185–90.
45. Zimmerli W, Trampuz A, Ochsner PE. Prosthetic-joint infections. N Engl J Med 2004;351(16):1645–54.
46. Zimmerli W. Prosthetic joint infection: diagnosis and treatment. Curr Infect Dis Rep 2000;2(5):377–9.

Fusion Following Failed Total Ankle Replacement

Markus Wünschel, MD, Priv.-Doz.[a],*, Ulf G. Leichtle, MD[a],
Carmen I. Leichtle, MD[a], Christian Walter, MD[a], Falk Mittag, MD[a],
Eva Arlt, MD[a], Andreas Suckel, MD, Priv.-Doz.[b]

KEYWORDS

- Ankle fusion • Revision surgery • Tibiotalar fusion • Tibiotalocalcaneal fusion
- Total ankle replacement

KEY POINTS

- After failed total ankle replacement tibiotalar and tibiotalocalcaneal fusions are established treatment options.
- Depending on the available bone stock autogenous or allogenic bone graft is necessary using the resected autogenous fibula, autogenous iliac crest, or allogenic femoral head.
- To achieve a rigid fixation for bone healing different devices can be used, such as screws, blade plates, combinations of the former, or retrograde intramedullary compression nailing systems.
- Rehabilitation is usually performed with a period of partial weightbearing in an ankle-foot orthosis or short leg cast postoperative followed by increasing load depending on intraoperative stability and radiologic progress of the fusion.
- The available literature of the clinical results indicates that outcome of fusion after failed total ankle replacement partly depends on the patient's underlying diagnosis.

INTRODUCTION

Fusions have a long tradition in foot and ankle surgery. Even before the development of modern osteosynthesis material, fusions were performed. Because of lack of internal or external stabilization only using cast for stability, the rate of nonunion was high, often associated with long-lasting suffering for patients.[1,2] With the use of modern osteosynthesis techniques a fairly safe fusion can be achieved if basic principles are considered.

Unlike at most other regions of the body, in foot and ankle surgery fusion still represents the gold standard of surgical therapy. Up until now, apart from the ankle joint

[a] Department of Orthopaedic Surgery, University Hospital Tübingen, Hoppe-Seyler-Street 3, Tübingen 72076, Germany; [b] Department of Orthopaedics and Trauma Surgery, Klinikum Stuttgart, Katharinenhospital, Kriegsbergstrasse 60, Stuttgart 70174, Germany
* Corresponding author.
E-mail address: markus.wuenschel@uni-tuebingen.de

Clin Podiatr Med Surg 30 (2013) 187–198
http://dx.doi.org/10.1016/j.cpm.2012.10.009
0891-8422/13/$ – see front matter © 2013 Elsevier Inc. All rights reserved.

podiatric.theclinics.com

with good long-term results,[3] joint replacement has not been established in foot and ankle surgery. The reason for this is that the tarsal joints, in comparison with other major joints of the body, only have a very limited mobility,[4,5] so that fusion in the foot and ankle, depending on the location, usually only means a minimal restriction for the patient. Quite the contrary, stability and possibility of mostly pain-free movement is appreciated by patients. For years, the treatment of end-stage osteoarthritis of the ankle has been controversially discussed.[6–11] Ankle fusion is an established surgical procedure that leads to a loss of joint function and in the long-term is associated with ongoing degeneration in adjacent joints endangering clinical outcome.[12–14] For total ankle replacement promising results have been published.[15–17]

Two main causes for failure of total ankle replacement are aseptic loosening and infection.[16] Before revision surgery is performed, it is crucial that a potential infection be ruled out. In many cases the infection can only be stopped by definite removal of the implant and a fusion.

Many factors have been identified that make patients more susceptible to an infection. Diseases, such as diabetes mellitus, obesity, renal failure, rheumatoid arthritis, neoplasms, hemophilia,[18–21] and certain medications, such as cortisone or other immunosuppressive medication, lead to higher infection rates.[22]

The first step to initiate the right treatment is the correct diagnosis, which in this special entity is sometimes difficult to achieve because there is no single evidentiary symptom, diagnostic test, or imaging modality. If an aspiration is performed the causative agent can be isolated ideally, leading to a specific antibiotic therapy even before surgical treatment. The leukocyte count in the sample is another piece in completing the diagnostic process. Even though a preoperative aspiration might be sterile intraoperative swabs and tissue samples, especially of the periprosthetic membrane, need to be taken.[23–25] Histopathologic examination[26] and polymerase chain reaction screening tests for bacterial DNA have also been established to verify a prosthetic infection with the clear disadvantage that the results are available only postoperatively. When it comes to treatment there are several options. In short-lasting infections after primary total ankle replacement, chances are good to preserve the implant.[27] However, in the case of a chronic infection the bacteria has colonized the implant, which usually makes it necessary to remove it to control the infection. The acute hematogenous type of infection may happen years after primary total ankle replacement. In these cases an attempt to maintain the implant might be made if the implant and the bone stock are intact and clinical symptoms are acute.

The special situation in total ankle replacement compared with total knee replacement and total hip replacement is the scarce bone stock of the talus, diminished talar vascular perfusion, minimal soft tissue coverage, and creation of iatrogenic malleolar fractures. In many cases revision total ankle replacement cannot be performed because of massive loosening and bone loss. In these cases autogenous or allogenic bone graft is necessary using resected autogenous fibula, autogenous iliac crest, or allogenic femoral head to impede leg length differences. If a flat implant had been used and after removal there is enough bone to securely fixate the screws/blade, a tibiotalar fusion can be performed.[28] This option usually leads to loss of some leg length, which has to be communicated with the patient before surgery. In many cases, however, the talus alone cannot be used for the arthrodesis and needs either to be removed or reconstructed with bone graft. In these cases a tibiotalocalcaneal fusion is recommended. Osteosynthesis implants, such as blade plates or retrograde intramedullary compression nails, are appropriate forms of fixation in these settings.[29–31]

SURGICAL TECHNIQUE
Preoperative Planning

First, the decision between an isolated tibiotalar fusion or a tibiotalocalcaneal fusion has to be made. From the authors experience, in most cases a tibiotalocalcaneal fusion is required because of talar bone loss as shown in **Fig. 1**. Their preferred method of osteosynthesis is a retrograde intramedullary compression nail. The foot and ankle have to be clinically and radiologically evaluated and other possible deformities that might be present need to be addressed, namely deformities of the hindfoot (**Fig. 2**). Therefore, a weightbearing hindfoot alignment radiograph including the calcaneus, ankle, and the lower leg is useful. Here the surgeon can detect deformities and can template the approximate diameter and length of implant to use. The clinical work-up also needs to include a vascular examination to rule out a disturbed blood flow. If this is disregarded major wound and bone healing complications can occur, which might necessitate plastic surgery coverage or amputation. The patient needs to be informed about potential need for autogenous bone graft harvesting and transplantation; possible adjacent joint degeneration; leg length discrepancy; general surgical risks, such as infection, bleeding, hematoma, nerve damage, nonunion, or malunion; peri-implant fracture; implant failure; and further revision surgery.

Preparation and Patient Positioning

The patient is typically positioned in a supine position (depending on the nailing system). The ipsilateral thigh is elevated by a cushion for better access to the lateral part of the ankle, which should overhang the operating table by approximately 15 cm. This is necessary for easier use of the targeting device and posteroanterior screw placement. The contralateral leg should be lowered down a few centimeters on a separate arm-board that simplifies use of the intraoperative image intensification

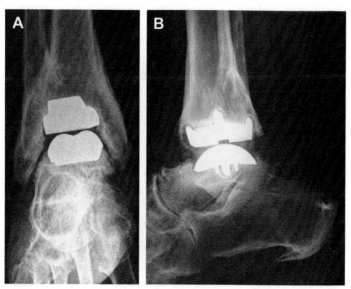

Fig. 1. Anteroposterior (A) and lateral (B) radiographs of a 55-year-old female patient 2 years after primary total ankle replacement performed because of posttraumatic ankle arthritis. Loosening and subsidence of the tibial and talar component are obvious. The talar body is markedly diminished and cannot be used for an isolated tibiotalar fusion.

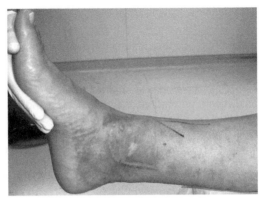

Fig. 2. Clinical presentation of the patient revealing multiple scarring after previous surgeries and a considerable equinus contracture that needs to be corrected.

C-arm. A tourniquet is applied at the thigh and inflated after inducing an Esmarch ischemia. In patients with expected extended duration of surgery or known vascular problems (eg, arterial conclusion disease), a tourniquet should not be used. After preparing the patient the leg is draped up to the thigh covering the tourniquet but leaving the knee joint in the operating field. This is important because the patella is an important guide for ultimate foot and ankle alignment.

SURGICAL APPROACH

The standard approach is an anterolateral skin incision starting approximately 8 cm above the tip of the lateral malleolus reaching down to the subtalar joint and then, curving forward, ending at the sinus tarsi. With this approach the fibula, ankle, and subtalar joint can be exposed (**Fig. 3**).

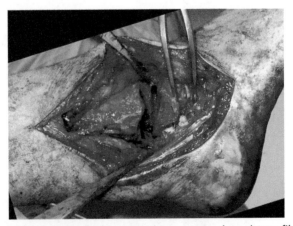

Fig. 3. Intraoperative photograph demonstrating an anterolateral transfibular approach. The fibula has been osteotomized and removed; the Hohmann-retractors open up the ankle joint, which has a large osseous defect caused by talar bone loss. The arthrodesis spreader is positioned in the subtalar joint. The peroneal tendons are visible and are protected by Hohmann-retractors.

Surgical Procedure

After the fibula has been exposed, the periosteum is split and stripped of the bone. The fibula is thereafter osteotomized approximately 6 cm above the tibiotalar joint line. After transecting the syndesmosis, the osteotomized distal fibula can be removed and stored in a saline-moistened compress for later use. Now a free vision of the joint is feasible and the implants of the total ankle replacement can be removed using a chisel, bone hook, or broad periosteal elevator. During this step the surgeon must be aware that only as much bone as necessary should be removed, always keeping in mind the already scarce bone stock of the talus (**Fig. 4**). After this is completed, a thorough debridement, synovectomy, and irrigation are indicated followed by removal of necrotic bone until healthy bone is reached (**Boxes 1** and **2**).[32–38] If an infection is suspected, intraoperative swabs should be taken with the implant in place and immediately after removal. Parts of the periprosthetic membrane should also be sent for microbiologic and histopathologic examination. In case of infection there are several ways to continue treatment, such as negative pressure wound therapy, primary septic fusion with external fixation, or temporary treatment with a polymethyl-methacrylate antibiotic loaded spacer or beads. In these cases an intramedullary nail should only be used after proved eradication of the infection by joint aspirate 6 weeks after removal of the implants.

Next, the subtalar joint needs be addressed. Using an arthrodesis spreader, the joint is dilated opened and the cartilage and sclerotic bone is completely removed with hand instrumentation. Various shaped chisels simplify this step of the procedure. After the ankle and the subtalar joints have been prepared, it is time to decide how to fill the osseous gap present. In many situations, the distal fibula is sufficient because it can be cut in several pieces of bicortical bone graft of the desired length. If the gap is too large, autogenous bone should be harvested from the iliac crest or a femoral head allograft can be used. Regardless of bone graft type, the entire defect across the ankle and subtalar joint surfaces should be packed with bone graft compressed into place.

The plantar insertion point of the nail is marked with a pen using an intraoperative image intensifier and a radiopaque metal rod. In addition to topographic landmarks,[39] the use of lateral and an axial image of the ankle/calcaneus allows a precise mark of the ideal entry point of the nail. The skin incision is made longitudinally at the point of the two crossing lines and extends 2 cm in each direction. Blunt dissection is carried

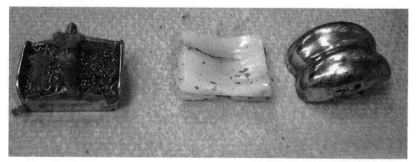

Fig. 4. Photograph of the explanted failed total ankle replacement. From left to right, superior surface of the tibial tray, talar articulating side of the ultrahigh molecular weight polyethylene insert, and superior surface of the talar component. Note the severe wear of the ultrahigh molecular weight polyethylene insert.

Box 1
Frequent patient-related reasons for nonunion after joint fusions

- Nicotine abuse
- Alcohol abuse
- Osteonecrosis of the talus
- Diabetes mellitus
- Psychiatric diseases
- Medication

Data from Refs.[33–36]

---

down to the calcaneus during which the plantar fascia usually has to be split and the neurovascular bundle needs to be protected medially. After inserting the guide sleeve a guidewire is inserted into the calcaneus through the talus proximally into the distal tibial shaft. Now the image intensification C-arm is used to verify the correct position of the guidewire and the ankle and hindfoot alignment in orthogonal planes. Thereafter, sequential reaming is performed either by hand, or more commonly with power reamers. An overreaming of 0.5 to 1 mm is recommended for easier nail insertion and to limit iatrogenic tibial fracture. The nail is mounted on the target device and inserted over the guidewire. Image intensification control of correct insertion depth of the nail is performed. Most of the available nails for tibiotalocalcaneal fusion are anatomically designed for this location; thus, the surgeon needs to take care to insert the nail in the correct position. After the nail, the ankle, and the hindfoot are positioned, the locking screws are inserted and compression performed. The way this is performed varies widely depending on the type of nail used.[32] The authors use the T2 ankle arthrodesis nailing system (Stryker Trauma, Schönkirchen, Germany), which allows selective compression of the ankle and the subtalar joints. Briefly, for this system after placing the talar locking screw in an oblong hole and placing the two proximal tibial screws, the harvested bone graft is positioned into the ankle joint around the nail. Now the internal compression screw, which has been preloaded inside the nail, is turned clockwise thus pushing the distal transverse screw and creating tibiotalar compression. The surgeon needs to take care that the talar screw does not cut through the bone or causes a fracture especially in osteoporotic bone (**Fig. 5**). Now talocalcaneal compression can be induced by applying external compression with an apposition ring against the plantar heel. Subsequently, two calcaneal locking screws are placed,

---

Box 2
Frequent surgery-related reasons for nonunion after joint fusions

- Infection
- Inadequate osteosynthesis
- Insufficient preparation of the bone surfaces
- Wrong alignment of the arthrodesis
- Inadequate postoperative treatment

Data from Refs.[34,37,38]

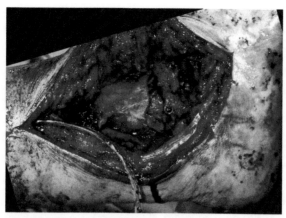

Fig. 5. Intraoperative photograph after inserting and locking the retrograde intramedullary nail. Just above the screw head of the talar locking screw the bicortical fibula autografts are visible. A wound drain has also been inserted.

one from lateral and one from posterior. Now the target device can be removed and an end cap is inserted. Final intraoperative image intensification C-arm is performed. Special attention has to be paid to the posteroanterior calcaneal locking screw. Because of its long course through bone, this screw might not pass though the nail, although the target device has been used (**Fig. 6**). Once proper screw placement is verified, the surgical sites are irrigated, a deep suction drain is inserted, and the incisions are closed in layers. The authors then apply a sterile compression dressing and deflate the tourniquet. In long cases the tourniquet should be deflated in intervals or not be used at all.

IMMEDIATE POSTOPERATIVE CARE

A split below-the-knee cast is applied in the operating room. The patient is mobilized without weightbearing after 2 days of bed rest. At this time the drain is removed and a dressing change made. Once the swelling goes down a circular cast with an anterior cutout window is placed. The patient usually is discharged 5 to 7 days after surgery.

REHABILITATION AND RECOVERY

The sutures are removed 14- to 21-days postoperative. After 6 weeks of nonweight-bearing the cast is removed and radiographs obtained. Then a new circular cast or pneumatic boot is applied and depending on the degree of consolidation, the patient usually is allowed to bear weight as tolerated. As long as the cast or boot is worn deep venous thrombosis prophylaxis is performed. Only in rare cases with signs of decelerated bone healing do the authors dynamize the nail by removing the static proximal tibia screw. After a total of 12-weeks postoperative another radiograph is taken and if osseous consolidation is verified the patient may walk freely. Hardware removal is reserved only for young patients or those who complain about pain and is performed at the earliest 6-months postoperative and when the joints are verified to be completely fused (**Fig. 7**). If necessary, the patient gets a prescription for orthopedic shoe wear with a rocker-bottom sole and insoles.

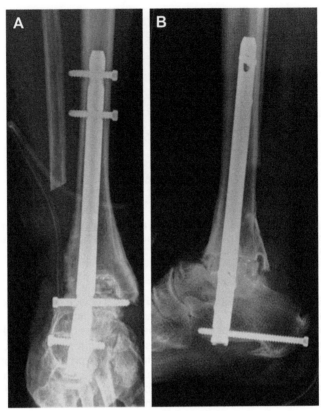

Fig. 6. Immediately postoperative anteroposterior (*A*) and lateral (*B*) radiographs. Leg length was maintained using the fibula interposition autografts, which can be well recognized. Also visible are some metal artifacts representing the remains of the former prosthesis. The retrograde intramedullary nail has built-in 5 degree of valgus in the frontal plane; the ankle was brought into neutral position in the sagittal plane.

CLINICAL RESULTS IN THE LITERATURE

The literature concerning this topic is limited. Only a few series with more than 20 patients have been published. Often case reports[40] and surgical techniques[41–43] have been published. Zarutsky and colleagues[44] retrospectively reviewed 43 cases of salvage ankle arthrodesis with a circular wire external fixation. Eighty percent of the patients had a solid fusion and 68.3% had a good result. Kitaoka and Romness[45] also describe their results for arthrodesis after failed total ankle replacement. Using four different fusion techniques their union rate was 89%. A total of 80% of the patients had no or mild pain.

Pelton and colleagues[46] report their results with salvage ankle arthrodesis using an intramedullary nail. Of 33 consecutively tibiotalocalcaneal procedures performed, 88% fused after a mean time of 3.7 months. Arthrodesis of the ankle secondary to replacement was also examined by Calsson and colleagues.[47] Of 100 total ankle replacements, 21 failed (16 of which suffered from rheumatoid arthritis). Seventeen of the 21 failed total ankle replacements fused using a Hoffman external fixator.

Carlsson[48] also describes a technical failure using a titanium mesh as interposition. None of the three treated ankles fused. However, Henricson and Rydholm[49] reported

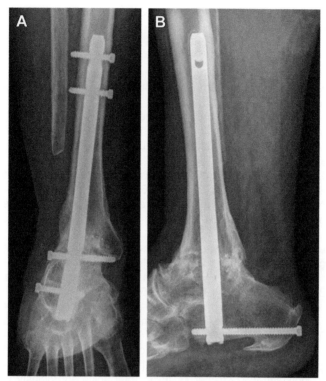

Fig. 7. One-year postoperative anteroposterior (*A*) and lateral (*B*) radiographs demonstrating mature osseous consolidation without complications.

good results after inserting a trabecular metal implant to bridge the osseous defect. Seven of 13 patients were pain-free, five had some residual pain, and one patient was dissatisfied.

Berkowitz and colleagues[50] published their results of tibiotalar and tibiotalocalcaneal fusion after failed total ankle replacement. They identified subtalar nonunion as a primary risk and advised a separate approach to prepare the subtalar joint for fusion. Kotnis and colleagues[51] report about 16 patients after failed ankle replacement, 14 of those caused by aseptic loosening. Five patients could be treated by revision total ankle replacement and nine with a fusion; clinical data were not disclosed. Fifteen out of 16 patients were treated successfully with tibiotalar fusion by Culpan and colleagues.[52] The one patient who did not fuse suffered from rheumatoid arthritis. Doets and Zurcher[53] analyzed a patient collective of 18 patients (15 patients had inflammatory joint disease) and revealed that inflammatory joint disease led to a significantly higher nonunion rate compared with other diagnosis. Blade plate fixation was the most successful type of osteosynthesis in this series. Hopgood and colleagues[54] had 17 unions in 23 patients treated by different types of procedures. The complication rate was again noted to be higher in patients with rheumatoid arthritis.

SUMMARY

Tibiotalar and tibiotalocalcaneal fusions are valuable options in case of failed total ankle replacement. If basic principles during preoperative planning and surgery are followed, the patient benefits from these procedures with a clear improvement in health-related quality of life.

REFERENCES

1. Goldthwait JE. An operation for the stiffening of the ankle joint in infantile paralysis. Am J Orthop Surg 1908;5:271.
2. Ogston A. On flat-foot, and its cure by operation. BMJ 1884;1:110–1.
3. Gougoulias N, Khanna A, Maffulli N. How successful are current ankle replacements? A systematic review of the literature. Clin Orthop Relat Res 2010;468: 199–208.
4. Astion DJ, Deland JT, Otis JC, et al. Motion of the hindfoot after simulated arthrodesis. J Bone Joint Surg Am 1997;79:241–6.
5. Wülker N, Stukenborg C, Savory KM, et al. Hindfoot motion after isolated and combined arthrodeses: measurements in anatomic specimens. Foot Ankle Int 2000;21:921–7.
6. Eichinger S, Forst R, Kindervater M. Indications and alternatives for arthroplasty in young patients. Orthopade 2007;36:311–24 [in German].
7. Morgan CD, Henke JA, Bailey RW, et al. Long-term results of tibiotalar arthrodesis. J Bone Joint Surg Am 1985;67:546–50.
8. Stengel D, Bauwens K, Ekkernkamp A, et al. Efficacy of total ankle replacement with meniscal-bearing devices: a systematic review and meta-analysis. Arch Orthop Trauma Surg 2005;125:109–19.
9. Trieb K, Wirtz DC, Durr HR, et al. Results of arthrodesis of the upper ankle joint. Z Orthop Ihre Grenzgeb 2005;143:222–6 [in German].
10. Schuh R, Hofstaetter J, Krismer M, et al. Total ankle arthroplasty versus ankle arthrodesis. Comparison of sports, recreational activities and functional outcome. Int Orthop 2012;36:1207–14.
11. Haddad SL, Coetzee JC, Estok R, et al. Intermediate and long-term outcomes of total ankle arthroplasty and ankle arthrodesis. A systematic review of the literature. J Bone Joint Surg Am 2007;89:1899–905.
12. Ahlberg A, Henricson AS. Late results of ankle fusion. Acta Orthop Scand 1981; 52:103–5.
13. Coester LM, Saltzman CL, Leupold J, et al. Long-term results following ankle arthrodesis for post-traumatic arthritis. J Bone Joint Surg Am 2001;83-A:219–28.
14. Hendrickx RP, Stufkens SA, de Bruijn EE, et al. Medium- to long-term outcome of ankle arthrodesis. Foot Ankle Int 2011;32:940–7.
15. Valderrabano V, Pagenstert G, Horisberger M, et al. Sports and recreation activity of ankle arthritis patients before and after total ankle replacement. Am J Sports Med 2006;34:993–9.
16. Krause FG, Windolf M, Bora B, et al. Impact of complications in total ankle replacement and ankle arthrodesis analyzed with a validated outcome measurement. J Bone Joint Surg Am 2011;93:830–9.
17. Guyer AJ, Richardson G. Current concepts review: total ankle arthroplasty. Foot Ankle Int 2008;29:256–64.
18. Dowsey MM, Choong PF. Obese diabetic patients are at substantial risk for deep infection after primary total knee arthroplasty. Clin Orthop Relat Res 2009;467: 1577–81.
19. Lubbeke A, Moons KG, Garavaglia G, et al. Outcomes of obese and non-obese patients undergoing revision total hip arthroplasty. Arthritis Rheum 2008;59: 738–45.

20. Namba RS, Paxton L, Fithian DC, et al. Obesity and peri-operative morbidity in total hip and total knee arthroplasty patients. J Arthroplasty 2005;20:46–50.
21. Lentino JR. Prosthetic joint infections: bane of orthopedists, challenge for infectious disease specialists. Clin Infect Dis 2003;36:1157–61.
22. Pietsch M, Wenisch C, Hofmann S. Treatment of infected total knee arthroplasty. 2-5-year results following two-stage re-implantation. Orthopade 2009;38:348–54 [in German].
23. Haddad FS, Muirhead-Allwood SK, Manktelow AR, et al. Two-stage uncemented revision hip arthroplasty for infection. J Bone Joint Surg Br 2000;82:689–94.
24. Lohmann CH, Furst M, Niggemeyer O, et al. The treatment of periprosthetic infections. Z Rheumatol 2007;66:28–33 [in German].
25. Bauer TW, Parvizi J, Kobayashi N, et al. Diagnosis of periprosthetic infection. J Bone Joint Surg Am 2006;88:869–82.
26. Morawietz L, Classen RA, Schroder JH, et al. Proposal for a histopathological consensus classification of the periprosthetic interface membrane. J Clin Pathol 2006;59:591–7.
27. Giulieri SG, Graber P, Ochsner PE, et al. Management of infection associated with total hip arthroplasty according to a treatment algorithm. Infection 2004; 32:222–8.
28. Kitaoka HB. Fusion techniques for failed total ankle arthroplasty. Semin Arthroplasty 1992;3:51–7.
29. Anderson T, Linder L, Rydholm U, et al. Tibio-talocalcaneal arthrodesis as a primary procedure using a retrograde intramedullary nail: a retrospective study of 26 patients with rheumatoid arthritis. Acta Orthop 2005;76:580–7.
30. Schill S. Ankle arthrodesis with interposition graft as a salvage procedure after failed total ankle replacement. Oper Orthop Traumatol 2007;19:547–60 [in German].
31. Wapner KL. Salvage of failed and infected total ankle replacements with fusion. Instr Course Lect 2002;51:153–7.
32. Thomas RL, Sathe V, Habib SI. The use of intramedullary nails in tibiotalocalcaneal arthrodesis. J Am Acad Orthop Surg 2012;20:1–7.
33. Cobb TK, Gabrielsen TA, Campbell DC, et al. Cigarette smoking and nonunion after ankle arthrodesis. Foot Ankle Int 1994;15:64–7.
34. Easley ME, Trnka HJ, Schon LC, et al. Isolated subtalar arthrodesis. J Bone Joint Surg Am 2000;82:613–24.
35. Mann RA, Rongstad KM. Arthrodesis of the ankle: a critical analysis. Foot Ankle Int 1998;19:3–9.
36. Perlman MH, Thordarson DB. Ankle fusion in a high-risk population: an assessment of nonunion risk factors. Foot Ankle Int 1999;20:491–6.
37. Cooper PS. Complications of ankle and tibiotalocalcaneal arthrodesis. Clin Orthop Relat Res 2001;391:33–44.
38. Mäenpää H, Lehto MU, Belt EA. What went wrong in triple arthrodesis? An analysis of failures in 21 patients. Clin Orthop Relat Res 2001;391:218–23.
39. Roukis TS. Determining the insertion site for retrograde intramedullary nail fixation of tibiotalocalcaneal arthrodesis: a radiographic and intraoperative anatomical analysis. J Foot Ankle Surg 2008;45:227–34.
40. Johl C, Kircher J, Pohlmannn K, et al. Management of failed total ankle replacement with a retrograde short femoral nail: a case report. J Orthop Trauma 2006; 20:60–5.
41. Ritter M, Nickisch F, DiGiovanni C. Technique tip: posterior blade plate for salvage of failed total ankle arthroplasty. Foot Ankle Int 2006;27:303–4.

42. Thomason K, Eyres KS. A technique of fusion for failed total replacement of the ankle: tibio-allograft-calcaneal fusion with a locked retrograde intramedullary nail. J Bone Joint Surg Br 2008;90:885–8.

43. Schuberth JM, Christensen JC, Rialson JA. Metal-reinforced cement augmentation for complex talar subsidence in failed total ankle arthroplasty. J Foot Ankle Surg 2011;50:766–72.

44. Zarutsky E, Rush SM, Schuberth JM. The use of circular wire external fixation in the treatment of salvage ankle arthrodesis. J Foot Ankle Surg 2005;44:22–31.

45. Kitaoka HB, Romness DW. Arthrodesis for failed ankle arthroplasty. J Arthroplasty 1992;7:277–84.

46. Pelton K, Hofer JK, Thordarson DB. Tibiotalocalcaneal arthrodesis using a dynamically locked retrograde intramedullary nail. Foot Ankle Int 2006;27:759–63.

47. Carlsson AS, Montgomery F, Besjakov J. Arthrodesis of the ankle secondary to replacement. Foot Ankle Int 1998;19:240–5.

48. Carlsson A. Unsuccessful use of a titanium mesh cage in ankle arthrodesis: a report on three cases operated on due to a failed ankle replacement. J Foot Ankle Surg 2008;47:337–42.

49. Henricson A, Rydholm U. Use of a trabecular metal implant in ankle arthrodesis after failed total ankle replacement. Acta Orthop 2010;81:745–7.

50. Berkowitz MJ, Clare MP, Walling AK, et al. Salvage of failed total ankle arthroplasty with fusion using structural allograft and internal fixation. Foot Ankle Int 2011;32:S493–502.

51. Kotnis R, Pasapula C, Anwar F, et al. The management of failed ankle replacement. J Bone Joint Surg Br 2006;88:1039–47.

52. Culpan P, Le SV, Piriou P, et al. Arthrodesis after failed total ankle replacement. J Bone Joint Surg Br 2007;89:1178–83.

53. Doets HC, Zurcher AW. Salvage arthrodesis for failed total ankle arthroplasty. Acta Orthop 2010;81:142–7.

54. Hopgood P, Kumar R, Wood PL. Ankle arthrodesis for failed total ankle replacement. J Bone Joint Surg Br 2006;88:1032–8.

Tibio-talo-calcaneal Arthrodesis with Retrograde Compression Intramedullary Nail Fixation for Salvage of Failed Total Ankle Replacement: A Systematic Review

Michael P. Donnenwerth, DPM[a], Thomas S. Roukis, DPM, PhD[b],*

KEYWORDS

• Ankle replacement • Revision • Arthrodesis • Surgery

KEY POINTS

- A systematic review of the world literature reveals a nonunion rate of 24.2% for patients who undergo tibio-talo-calcaneal arthrodesis with retrograde compression intramedullary nail fixation for a failed total ankle replacement.
- Modified American Orthopaedic Foot and Ankle Society Ankle and Hindfoot Scale scores demonstrated fair patient outcomes of 58.1 points on an 86-point scale (67.6 points on a 100-point scale); however, these are satisfactory given the alternative to this procedure and fixation combination is amputation.
- Complications were observed in 38 of 62 (62.3%) patients reviewed, with the most common complication being nonunion.
- Failed total ankle replacement is a complex problem that should only be treated by experienced foot and ankle surgeons. Tibio-talo-calcaneal arthrodesis with retrograde compression intramedullary nail fixation offers a reliable option for failed total ankle replacement.

INTRODUCTION

Total ankle replacement has been used for severe ankle degenerative arthritis since the 1970s.[1–4] Early generations were fraught with problems and complications.[5–8] Revision replacement often resulted in unsatisfactory outcomes, and salvage

Financial Disclosure: None reported.
Conflict of Interest: None reported.
[a] Department of Orthopaedics, Section of Podiatry, Gundersen Lutheran Medical Foundation, Mail Stop C03-006A, 1836 South Avenue, La Crosse, WI 54601, USA; [b] Department of Orthopaedics, Podiatry, and Sports Medicine, Gundersen Lutheran Healthcare System, 2nd Floor Founders Building, Mail Stop FB2-009, 1900 South Avenue, La Crosse, WI 54601, USA
* Corresponding author.
E-mail address: tsroukis@gundluth.org

arthrodesis was the primary recommendation for a failed total ankle replacement.[5] Salvage fusion was often difficult with massive bone loss.[6] This finding lead many foot and ankle surgeons to conclude that arthrodesis may be a superior primary operation for severe degenerative arthritis of the ankle.[9,10] However, advances in technology used for components, as well as instrumentation have allowed total ankle replacement to regain popularity as an alternative to ankle arthrodesis.[11–15]

Despite the improved designs of current systems, some studies suggest that a steep learning curve exists with total ankle replacement.[16–18] As a result, postoperative complications and ultimately failures are inevitable. Postoperative complications leading to the need for revision include aseptic loosening with subsidence of components, deep peri-prosthetic infection, and wound-healing problems.[1–20] Revision involves removal and exchange of implant components, conversion to arthrodesis, or amputation of the leg.[19,20] Although revision with implant exchange is often possible, the extensive bone loss that can occur with subsidence of components may result in arthrodesis as the only feasible salvage option for a failed total ankle replacement.[21]

When revision total ankle replacement is not an option, and arthrodesis is the desired operative course, several decisions are required. Careful selection of fixation choice must be made given the complexity that exists with salvage arthrodesis for a failed total ankle replacement. Additionally, many patients with failed total ankle replacement have concomitant subtalar joint disease, and revision of the total ankle replacement with isolated ankle arthrodesis is not ideal. When the talus becomes cystic or collapsed from subsidence, tibio-talar arthrodesis can be extremely difficult, necessitating tibio-talo-calcaneal arthrodesis. Bone grafting is often necessary to fill the void left from the removed implant components in a failed total ankle replacement.[5,6,19,22–31]

Myriad fixation techniques can be employed including: combination screw and plate internal fixation alone, external fixation alone, combination internal and external fixation, as well as, retrograde compression intramedullary nail fixation.[21–30] When tibio-talo-calcaneal arthrodesis is necessary, a retrograde compression intramedullary nail provides reliable, reproducible fixation with external and/or internal compression and the option for dynamization postoperatively. Although retrograde compression intramedullary nail fixation has historically been considered to have high complication rates, a recent systematic review[31] that included 461 tibio-talo-calcaneal arthrodesis procedures for a variety of etiologies with a retrograde intramedullary nail revealed that most reoperations (70%) were for hardware removal. Nonunion was stated at 13.3% (85 of 641 cases); however, only 3.4% (22 of 641 cases) required revision arthrodesis. No prior study exists specifically evaluating the success of tibio-talo-calcaneal arthrodesis using retrograde compression intramedullary nail fixation specifically for failed total ankle replacement. Therefore, the authors conducted a systematic review of this topic.

MATERIALS AND METHODS

The authors performed a systematic review of electronic databases and relevant peer-reviewed sources including OvidSP-Medline (http://ovidsp.tx.ovid.com/; last accessed June 24, 2012) and a general scientific search engine (http://google.com; last accessed June 24, 2012). Additionally, the authors searched common American, British, and European orthopedic and podiatric medical journals for relevant manuscripts. Only manuscripts published in peer-reviewed journals that involved outcomes of a series greater than 5 tibio-talo-calcaneal arthrodesis procedures with the use of a retrograde compression intramedullary nail fixation for a failed total ankle replacement were included (**Fig. 1**).

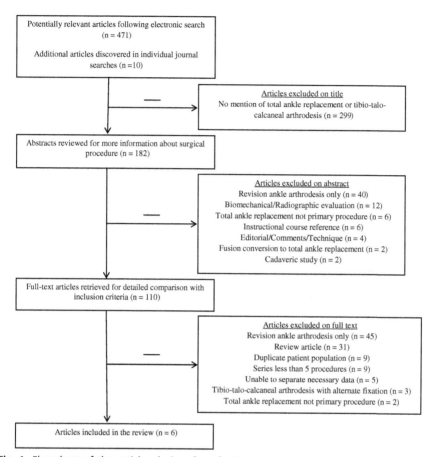

Fig. 1. Flowchart of the articles during the selection process.

The authors performed the systematic review with no restriction on date or language, using an inclusive text word query "failed" OR "failure" OR "revision" AND "total ankle" OR "tibio-talo-calcaneal," where the all upper-case words represent the boolean operators employed. Retrieved manuscript references were searched to identify additional potential articles for inclusion. Also, in situations where more information was needed regarding technique or patient outcome, the authors electronically contacted those authors requesting supplementary information. Consensus was employed for final inclusion, with the lead author (MPD) being the moderator.

RESULTS

The search for potentially eligible information yielded a total of 481 references (see **Fig. 1**). All references identified were obtained and reviewed by the authors in February 2012, and a second search was performed in May 2012 to determine if new articles existed; none were identified. After considering all potentially eligible references, 6 articles (1.2%) met the authors' inclusion criteria and were included in the present study.[22–27] All of the manuscripts were evidence-based medicine level 4 studies, involving small case series. Sixty-one patients with 62 failed total ankle replacements were included in this study. The weight mean age of patients provided was 58.8 years (range: 17–80-years). Of these patients, the original total ankle replacement system was provided in 56 patients (90.3%, 32 STAR, 12 Buechel-Pappas, 5 Thompson-Richards, 3 Bath and Wessex, 2 Imperial, and 1 Salto Tolaris).[22–26] After explantation of the failed total ankle replacement, bone grafting was required in 59 of 62 ankles (95.2%). Complications occurred in 38 of 62 patients (62.3%). These included: 15 (24.2%) nonunions, 6 (9.7%) superficial wound infections, 6 (9.7%) removal of painful or irritated hardware (excluding nail removal for revision of nonunions), 3 (4.9%) delayed unions, 3 (4.9%) deep infections, 2 (3.3%) nerve-related injuries, 2 (3.3%) tibial stress fractures, and 1 (1.6%) below-knee amputation.

Nonunion after the initial salvage tibio-talo-calcaneal arthrodesis occurred in 15 of 62 ankles (24.2%, 12 ankle and 3 subtalar joint nonunions). Revision arthrodesis was required in 9 patients (14.5%). The remaining nonunions were treated with bracing alone. The weighted mean follow-up was 25.8 months (range: 12–88 months) for the studies in which those data were included.[22–25,27] Outcomes were measured using the American Orthopaedic Foot and Ankle Society Ankle and Hindfoot Scale (AOFAS-AHS) with a maximum of 86 points for tibio-talo-calcaneal arthrodesis, given the loss of motion at the ankle and subtalar joints. The weighted mean postoperative score was 58.1 (range: 35–86) for studies that included this scoring scale.[22,25,26]

The methodological quality of the included studies was fair. All manuscripts included were level 4 studies. The patient populations were small, and often information had to be extrapolated from larger groups. All included manuscripts were published in peer-reviewed journals (**Table 1**).

DISCUSSION

The purpose of this systematic review was to determine the success of tibio-talo-calcaneal arthrodesis with retrograde compression intramedullary nail fixation for failed total ankle replacement. A total of 6 studies could be identified that met the authors' inclusion criteria. All studies described the operative intervention as removal of the failed implant components, use of bone graft, and tibio-talo-calcaneal arthrodesis with retrograde compression intramedullary nail fixation.[22–27] The surgical exposure did vary, although a lateral dissection with transfibular approach was often employed.[22–25] This afforded the surgeon access to both the ankle and subtalar joints to explant the failed total ankle replacement and prepare the joints for arthrodesis through 1 primary incision with a smaller anterior medial incision used for complete joint preparation. Bone grafting was used in 59 of 62 ankles (95.2%), with a variety of autograft and allograft selections. The choice of bone graft did not appear to change the outcome.

AOFAS-AHS scores were used in 3 reviewed manuscripts and totaled a weighted mean of 58.1 on an 86-point scale (ie, 67.6 on a 100-point scale). The manuscripts had altered the scoring scale to account for the loss of subtalar and ankle motion. Although the AOFAS-AHS only equates to a fair overall outcome for these patients, this is acceptable given that the tibio-talo-calcaneal arthrodesis was often a revision of multiple failed attempts to correct the problematic ankle. With virtually no other procedure choice beyond amputation for a failed total ankle replacement that cannot undergo revision of implant components, the outcomes observed with this procedure and fixation option are satisfactory.

Nonunion was determined by lack of trabecular pattern, clinical motion present across the ankle or subtalar joint, or hardware failure. The present study demonstrated a 24.2% nonunion rate in patients undergoing tibio-talo-calcaneal arthrodesis with

Table 1
Statistical description of the studies that met the criteria for inclusion in the systematic review

Author (y) [Level of Evidence]	Total Number of Patients	Total Number of Ankles	Mean Age (y) [Range]	Mean Follow up (mo) [Range]	Number of Nonunions (%)	Complications	Mean Postoperative AOFAS-AHS [Range]
Anderson et al,[22] (2005) [4]	15	16	62 [17–82]	34 [15–88]	5/16 (31.5)	13	56.7 [40–80]
Hopgood et al,[23] (2006) [4]	10	10	N/A	N/A	2/10 (20)	5	N/A
Kotniz et al,[24] (2006) [4]	9	9	N/A	12	0/9 (0)	0	N/A
Schill,[25] (2007) [4]	15	15	56 [46–76]	23 [7–36]	1/15 (6.7)	7	57.9 [35–81]
Doets and Zurcher,[26] (2010) [4]	6	6	58 [43–76]	N/A	4/6 (66.7)	6	62 [38–86]
Berkowitz et al,[27] (2011) [4]	6	6	N/A	33.2 [12–80]	3/6 (50)	7	N/A
Totals	61	62	32.6 [15–64]	25.8 [7–88]	15/62 (24.2)	38	58.1 [35–86]

Abbreviations: F, female; M, male; N/A, not available.

retrograde compression intramedullary nail fixation for failed total ankle replacement. This number is relatively high, compared with an article by Jehan and colleagues.[32] They recently published a systematic review on the success of tibio-talo-calcaneal arthrodesis using retrograde compression intramedullary nail fixation and found a nonunion rate of 13.3% (85 of 641 cases). The comparison between these nonunion rates lends to the difficulty to achieve union in a tibio-talo-calcaneal arthrodesis for patients with a failed total ankle replacement as patients with other ankle pathology have a significantly lower nonunion rate.[32] One series of patients reviewed was treated strictly with an anterior incision.[27] Of the 6 patients extrapolated from this article, 3 developed a nonunion. The authors described that the subtalar joint was not formally débrided in the 3 cases of nonunion. The subtalar joint had been accessed from the same primary anterior incision. Revision was performed through a dedicated lateral incision, and all went on to solid arthrodesis. Although this is a small cohort of patients, one could infer that the anterior approach without lateral subtalar joint preparation should be avoided when performing tibio-talo-calcaneal arthrodesis for failed total ankle replacement with retrograde compression intramedullary nail fixation.

Complications occurred in 38 of 62 (62.3%) ankles reviewed. Jehan and colleagues[32] described the largest proportion of complications as related to metalwork (16.8%), which ultimately led to greater than half of their reviewed reoperations. Nonunion did comprise the second most common complication found, however (13.3%). In the present study, 21 of 38 (55.3%) of the complications observed were major. These included: 15 nonunions, 3 deep infections requiring removal of the nail, 2 tibial stress fractures, and 1 below-knee amputation. Metalwork-related complications were relatively small in number, occurring in 6 of 38 cases (15.8%). This finding again indicates that tibio-talo-calcaneal arthrodesis for failed total ankle replacement is a very complex process and that, like primary total ankle replacement, it should only be undertaken by foot and ankle surgeons experienced in performing these procedures.

The weaknesses of the present study include the fact that the search for pertinent references that met the authors' inclusion criteria was performed through electronic databases. It is possible that additional information may have been inadvertently overlooked or excluded. However, the number of references identified in the authors' search was quite high at 481, and each reference was carefully reviewed for possible inclusion. The inclusion criteria were very specific as well. This led to a number of references with patients who underwent this procedure being excluded, because the data were incomplete or mixed with other procedures. The authors attempted to contact the authors electronically on several occasions without response. In 1 instance,[33] a response was obtained regarding patients in their cohort; however, this information was excluded, as less than 5 tibio-talo-calcaneal arthrodesis procedures were detailed. Additionally, the inclusion of manuscripts with 5 or more procedures was arbitrary. The authors would have ideally liked to include only articles with greater than 10 tibio-talo-calcaneal arthrodesis procedures to reach the needed numbers to reliably assess for nonunion in this patient population. However, in doing so, the numbers included in the review would have been much lower (41 total procedures). To increase the odds of capturing meaningful numbers, the authors selected a procedure minimum of 5. This eliminated case studies from the potentially relevant references, which was desired. Additionally, different total ankle replacement systems, indications for primary total ankle replacement, type of bone graft employed, and specific retrograde compression intramedullary nail all reduce the generalization of this systematic review.

After a systematic review of peer-reviewed data, the success of tibio-talo-calcaneal arthrodesis with retrograde compression intramedullary nail fixation for failed total ankle replacement is consistent with a weighted mean AOFAS-AHS score of 58.1 points on a modified scale of 86 points. Nonunion occurred in 15 of 62 ankles (24.2%). Of these patients, 9 revision arthrodeses (14.5%) were performed, with the remaining obtaining stable pseudoarthroses and treated nonoperatively with bracing. Only 1 below-knee amputation was required. The high rate of complications and nonunion indicates that revision total ankle replacement and even isolated ankle fusion would be preferred to tibio-talo-calcaneal arthrodesis. However, in patients with massive bone loss secondary to failed total ankle replacement, retrograde compression intramedullary nail fixation for tibio-talo-calcaneal arthrodesis provides foot and ankle surgeons a viable option for salvage. Nevertheless, the world literature is limited with regard to this procedure choice and fixation combination. Further prospective studies comparing isolated ankle to tibio-talo-calcaneal arthrodesis as well as internal fixation constructs employing plate-and-screw constructs and retrograde compression intramedullary nail fixation should be undertaken.

REFERENCES

1. Lord G, Marotte JH. Total ankle prosthesis. Technique and 1st results. Apropos of 12 cases. Rev Chir Orthop Reparatrice Appar Mot 1973;59(2):139–51.
2. Stauffer RN. Total ankle joint replacement as an alternative to arthrodesis. Geriatrics 1976;31(3):79–82.
3. Pappas M, Beuchel FF, DePalma AF. Cylindrical total ankle replacement: surgical and biomechanical rationale. Clin Orthop Relat Res 1976;118:82–92.
4. Evanski PH, Waugh TR. Management of arthritis of the ankle. An alternative to arthrodesis. Clin Orthop Relat Res 1977;122:110–5.
5. Stauffer RN. Salvage of painful total ankle arthroplasty. Clin Orthop Relat Res 1982;170:184–8.
6. Kitaoka HB. Fusion techniques for failed total ankle arthroplasty. Semin Arthroplasty 1992;3(1):51–7.
7. Kitaoka HB, Patzer GL, Ilstrup DM, et al. Survivorship analysis of the Mayo total ankle arthroplasty. J Bone Joint Surg Am 1994;76(7):974–9.
8. Wynn AH, Wilde AH. Long-term follow-up of the Conaxial (Beck-Steffee) total ankle arthroplasty. Foot Ankle 1992;13(6):303–6.
9. Kirkup J. Richards Smith ankle arthroplasty. J R Soc Med 1984;78(4):301–4.
10. Bolton-Maggs BG, Sudlow RA, Freeman MA. Total ankle arthroplasty. A long-term review of the London Hospital experience. J Bone Joint Surg Br 1985;67(5): 785–90.
11. Nunley JA, Caputo AM, Easley ME, et al. Intermediate to long-term outcomes of the STAR total ankle replacement: the patient perspective. J Bone Joint Surg Am 2012;94(1):43–8.
12. Schuberth JM, McCourt MJ, Christensen JC. Interval changes in postoperative range of motion of Salto-Tolaris total ankle replacement. J Foot Ankle Surg 2011;50(5):562–5.
13. Schenk K, Lieske S, John M, et al. Prospective study of a cementless, mobile-bearing, third generation total ankle prosthesis. Foot Ankle Int 2011;32(8):755–63.
14. Buechel FF Sr. Evolution of the Buechel-Pappas mobile-bearing total ankle replacement. Foot Ankle Spec 2008;1(6):363–7.
15. Hintermann B, Valderrabano B, Knupp M, et al. The HINTEGRA ankle: short- and mid-term results. Orthopade 2006;35(5):533–45.
16. Murnaghan JM, Warnock DS, Henderson SA. Total ankle replacement. Early experience with STAR prosthesis. Ulster Med J 2005;74(1):9–13.

17. Lee KB, Cho SG, Hur CI, et al. Perioperative complications of HINTEGRA total ankle replacement. Our initial 50 cases. Foot Ankle Int 2008;29(10):978–84.
18. Lee KT, Lee YK, Young KW, et al. Perioperative complications of the Mobility total ankle system: comparison with HINTEGRA total ankle system. J Orthop Sci 2010; 15(3):317–22.
19. Henricson A, Carlsson A, Rydholm U. What is a revision of total ankle replacement? Foot Ankle Surg 2011;17:99–102.
20. Glazebrook MA, Arsenault K, Dunbar M. Evidence-based classification of complication in total ankle arthroplasty. Foot Ankle Int 2009;30:945–9.
21. Roukis TS. Incidence of revision after primary implantation of the Agility total ankle replacement system: a systematic review. J Foot Ankle Surg 2012;51: 198–204.
22. Anderson T, Rydholm U, Besjakov J, et al. Tibio-talo-calcaneal fusion using retrograde intramedullary nails as a salvage procedure for failed total ankle prostheses in rheumatoid arthritis: a report on sixteen cases. Foot Ankle Surg 2005; 11:143–7.
23. Hopgood P, Kumar R, Wood P. Ankle arthrodesis for failed total ankle replacement. J Bone Joint Surg Br 2006;88(8):1032–8.
24. Kotniz R, Pasapula C, Anwar F, et al. The management of failed ankle replacement. J Bone Joint Surg Br 2006;88(8):1039–47.
25. Schill S. Ankle arthrodesis with interposition graft as a salvage procedure after failed total ankle replacement. Oper Orthop Traumatol 2007;19(5):547–60.
26. Doets HC, Zurcher AW. Salvage arthrodesis for failed total ankle arthroplasty. Acta Orthop 2010;81(1):142–7.
27. Berkowitz MJ, Clare MP, Walling AK, et al. Salvage of failed total ankle arthroplasty with fusion using structural allograft and internal fixation. Foot Ankle Int 2011;32(5):493–502.
28. Fazal MA, Garrido E, Williams RL. Tibio-talo-calcaneal arthrodesis by retrograde intramedullary nail and bone grafting. Foot Ankle Surg 2006;12:185–90.
29. Pelton K, Hofer JK, Thordarson DB. Tibio-talo-calcaneal arthrodesis using a dynamically locked retrograde intramedullary nail. Foot Ankle Int 2006;27(10): 759–63.
30. Budnar VM, Hepple S, Harries WG, et al. Tibio-talo-calcaneal arthrodesis with a curved, interlocking, intramedullary nail. Foot Ankle Int 2010;31(12):1085–92.
31. Muckley T, Klos K, Drechsel T, et al. Short-term outcome of retrograde tibio-talo-calcaneal arthrodesis with a curved intramedullary nail. Foot Ankle Int 2011;32(1): 47–56.
32. Jehan S, Shakeel M, Bing A, et al. The success of tibio-talo-calcaneal arthrodesis with intramedullary nailing. A systematic review of the literature. Acta Orthop Belg 2011;77(5):644–51.
33. Hammett R, Heppple S, Forster B, et al. Tibio-talo-calcaneal (hindfoot) arthrodesis by retrograde intramedullary nailing using a curved locking nail. The results of 52 procedures. Foot Ankle Int 2005;26(10):810–5.

Failure of the Agility Total Ankle Replacement System and the Salvage Options

Graham McCollum, FCS Orth (SA), MD, Mark S. Myerson, MD*

KEYWORDS

- Arthroplasty • Agility • Joint pain • Joint replacement • Revision surgery

KEY POINTS

- Total ankle replacement is a demanding procedure that can ultimately fail for a variety of reasons and require revision. However, subsidence of the talus or tibia is the most common and the degree of subsidence has predictive value in determining revision possibilities and outcomes.
- Aseptic osteolysis is common in the first 2 years after implantation of the Agility total ankle replacement system, especially around the tibia. However, the degree of osteolysis should be minimal and not progress. Otherwise, failure can be expected over time.
- Cyst formation is common and should be treated at the time of revision with impaction bone grafting and only in select instances with polymethylmethacrylate cement.
- There are specific limitations to understand before attempting revision of a failed Agility total ankle replacement system. Considerations include revision talar component and UHMWPE inserts, LP tibial or talar components, custom stemmed tibial or talar components, and conversion to alternative total ankle replacement systems.
- A national joint arthroplasty registry data system is warranted, because this would provide useful information regarding survivorship of total ankle replacement.

INTRODUCTION

After the success of hip and knee arthroplasty, total ankle replacements were first attempted in the 1970s. Early outcomes were not encouraging because of the lack of understanding regarding ankle biomechanics, the bone-implant interface, and implant materials. These implants were usually cemented to the native bone, did not recreate the ankle anatomy or biomechanics, and were overconstrained. Early failure and poor patient satisfaction led to a trend in favor of arthrodesis over arthroplasty for end-stage ankle arthritis. Better understanding of tribiology and ankle

The Institute for Foot and Ankle Reconstruction, Mercy Medical Center, 301 Saint Paul Place, Baltimore, MD 21202, USA
* Corresponding author.
E-mail address: mark4feet@aol.com

Clin Podiatr Med Surg 30 (2013) 207–223
http://dx.doi.org/10.1016/j.cpm.2012.10.001
0891-8422/13/$ – see front matter © 2013 Published by Elsevier Inc.

podiatric.theclinics.com

mechanics led to renewed interest in total ankle replacement. Uncemented, less constrained implants together with improved surgical techniques and patient selection began to show encouraging results through the late 1980s. Implant survivorship and patient satisfaction have continued to improve, making total ankle replacement a viable and increasingly popular option.[1,2] The benefits of maintaining motion of the ankle joint are to provide a near normal gait profile and eliminate the incidence of adjacent joint arthritis. Unfortunately, total ankle replacement outcomes still remain inferior to that of the knee and hip and ongoing work and research are needed to improve this situation.[3] Failure can be the result of poor patient selection, poor surgical technique, postoperative infection, and implant-related factors.

Many total ankle replacement designs have entered the market over the past two decades with varying success. History has shown that enormous information and insight is gained from studying failures of an implant or surgical procedure. Throughout the world, joint replacement registries have yielded valuable information about implant survivorship and complications. They provide a nonbiased database for survivorship comparison and can detect early and late failures of prosthesese.[4] Recent identification of the adverse effects and catastrophic failure of metal-on-metal hip replacements was brought to the world's attention after study of international joint registries.[5] Unfortunately, enrollment of total ankle replacement into registries has not been as inclusive as the hip and the knee; only New Zealand, Norway, and Sweden document all primary and revision total ankle replacements. Better inclusion of total ankle replacement into registries is important and likely to yield valuable information in the future. Because this is not the case at present, retrospective studies, survival analysis, reporting of complications of an implant, and suggested salvage options would be valuable contributions to improving the procedure.

As more total ankle replacements are performed, more complications and situations requiring revision or reoperation will be encountered. The surgeon performing the primary procedure on a regular basis needs to understand failure patterns to try and prevent them in the first place, if possible, and also to detect them early enough so that surgical solutions are not limited. Sometimes the reasons for failure are technique- and surgeon-related but other times the implant itself is the causative factor. Performing revision total ankle replacement is complicated and ideally should be performed at an experienced specialist center where the necessary skills, knowledge, and equipment are available.

This article reviews the history of the development of the Agility total ankle replacement system (DePuy Orthopedics, Warsaw, IN) and illustrates certain complications specific to this implant, and other complications common to most total ankle replacement designs. Salvage options are discussed and examples from the senior author's (MSM) series are included.

HISTORY

The original Agility total ankle replacement system was designed and patented by Frank G. Alvine in the late 1970s but only came onto the market for selected surgeons in the United States in 1993. By 1999 it was made freely available to surgeons and soon became the most commonly implanted total ankle replacement in the United States.[6,7] There are more than 20 years of experience with the implant in this country and it has the longest follow-up data of a fixed-bearing device to date.[8] There have been several design modifications over the last 15 years, culminating in the fourth generation Agility currently available.[6,7]

The implant relies on distal tibiofibular syndesmosis arthrodesis to provide lateral support and bony ongrowth. The two-part prosthesis is semiconstrained with permissible medial-to-lateral translation and rotation of the talus under the ultrahigh molecular weight polyethylene (UHMWPE) insert. The design resurfaces not only the superior and inferior surfaces of the tibiotalar joint but also the medial and lateral recesses of the mortise. The first bearing surfaces were titanium on UHMWPE but poor wear characteristics of titanium led to the introduction of cobalt chrome for the talar component. Tibial base plate failure and fracture led to a thicker plate design, eliminating the complication of plate fracture and the posterior tibia was augmented to reduce posterior subsidence. The range of sizes was increased to six and a revision talus with a rectangular base plate was added. After study of failures and revision surgery, three more improvements to the implant were made and introduced in 2006: (1) a wider-based talar component with medial and lateral flanges to counteract subsidence (ie, Agility LP total ankle replacement system); (2) the ability to size-mismatch, improving modularity in revision circumstances; and (3) a front-loading UHMWPE insert mechanism for easier removal and insertion making exchange with a fixed tibial component much easier.[7] The difficulty of revision with earlier Agility models is illustrated in this article.

OUTCOME

Retrospective series' looking at Agility outcomes show good results initially, but this deteriorates with longer-term follow-up.[7] Pyevich and colleagues[9] reported on 100 of Alvinee's cases. At a mean follow-up of 4.8 years, there was a 6% revision rate but at 9-year follow-up of this same series and addition of another 32 cases by Knecht and colleagues[10] revealed that the revision rate increased to 11%. This seems to be comparable with outcomes of other prostheses, so some of the problems of the Agility are likely common to all total ankle replacement designs. Gougoulias and colleagues[11] reviewed the literature and included the results of 1105 total ankle replacements using six different prostheses' including the Agility total ankle replacement system and found no statistical difference in medium-term outcome. Similarly, Roukis[7] performed a systematic review and determined that the incidence of revision for the Agility total ankle replacement system was 9.7% (224 of 2312) at a weighted mean follow-up of 22.8 months.

Reoperation after total ankle replacement may include removal and replacement of the prosthesis or part thereof, osseous or soft tissue procedures, arthrodesis, and ablation. The Agility total ankle replacement implant has some specific complications that have been identified by the senior author since being first used in the mid-1990s. Other implants may have similar complications requiring revision but the focus of this article is on the Agility total ankle replacement system. Some of these indications are talar and tibial subsidence; aseptic loosening; cyst formation (symptomatic and asymptomatic); periprosthetic malleolar fracture; and syndesmotic nonunion. Other complications, such as arthrofibrosis and postoperative stiffness, wound dehiscence, and infection, common to all prostheses, are not discussed in this article.

The symptoms, cause, prevention, and treatment of each of these complications are discussed and illustrated and where possible surgical solutions suggested. The senior author has 15 years of experience with the Agility total ankle replacement system and its' subsequent generations of design, and because of the higher incidence of short- and long-term complications after its implantation, he has discontinued the use of this prosthesis for primary joint replacement.

CYST FORMATION

Bone loss surrounding an implant can lead to instability, loss of fixation, and subsidence. Data from hip and knee arthroplasty have revealed that wear, either of the UHMWPE insert or the metal surfaces of the bearing, generate particles that are distributed throughout the effective joint space. These particles, 100 to 500 μm (UHMWPE) in size, are able to track between the implant and the bone causing local osteolysis.[12] Osteoclastic recruitment, macrocyte-driven local histiocytic foreign body reaction, and inflammation are a reaction to these particles and lead to bone loss, loosening, or cyst formation.[13] Certain factors that increase UHMWPE wear are surgeon-dependent, such as poor alignment or rotation of an implant leading to abnormal contact stresses, and implant factors, such as the quality of the UHMWPE and certain mechanical factors of a particular prosthesis. For example, new-generation highly cross-linked ultralow molecular weight polyethylene is much more wear resistant than the conventional polyethylene first used by the Agility implant.[12] Vaupel and colleagues[14] looked at 10 failed Agility total ankle replacement implants and noted significant scratching, pitting, abrasion, and embedding of the UHMWPE with visible macroscopic erosion corresponding to the edges of the talar articulation. Titanium particles were found in the UHMWPE indicating third particle involvement, which is known to significantly increase wear.[12]

Periprosthetic cyst formation typically occurs on the tibial side, particularly in the medial malleolus and medial tibial plafond but also laterally when a nonunion of the syndesmosis has occurred.[9] These cysts may be asymptomatic initially if the implant remains well-supported and fixed or symptomatic with deep ankle and start-up pain (ie, pain worse when moving for the first time after a period of rest).

Radiographs can underrepresent the cyst because of intact anterior and posterior cortices, so computerized tomography (CT) scanning is mandatory to delineate the cystic anatomy and to determine the size and extent. The authors routinely obtain a CT scan when any patient presents with pain or dysfunction after implantation of the Agility total ankle replacement prosthesis (**Fig. 1**).

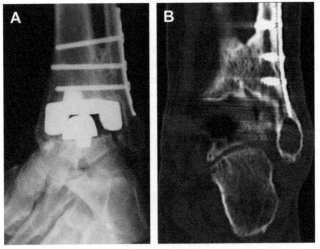

Fig. 1. Oblique radiograph (A) demonstrating a fibula cyst that is much larger on CT imaging (B).

Cysts appear up to three-times larger on CT compared with radiographs.[15] Radiographic features are periprosthetic lucency exceeding 2 mm or a lytic lesion in the distal tibial metaphysis. These should alert the clinician to the possibility of cyst formation.[9,15] CT scanning allows the percentage of tibial involvement and adjacent osteointegration to be determined to help decision making when it comes to planning revision surgery.

Treatment planning is challenging when an asymptomatic patient with a well-functioning total ankle replacement presents with a cyst. There is no foot and ankle literature to guide the decision to operate, but when cyst formation involves more than 50% of the weight-bearing surface of the acetabulum after hip replacement, stabilizing surgery with bone grafting and UHMWPE liner exchange in an asymptomatic patient is indicated.[16] This may be applicable to the distal tibia after total ankle replacement but speculative at this stage. If a small or moderate sized cyst is identified, serial CT scans and surveillance every 6 months to plot enlargement is mandatory to enable intervention before major bone loss, cortical destruction, and implant destabilization. Cysts are unpredictable; some remain quiescent or resolve[17] and do not destabilize the implant and continue to be asymptomatic, whereas others balloon and are destructive. Failure to note expansion and ballooning drastically changes the salvage options from bone grafting and UHMWPE insert exchange to a major revision requiring structural bone graft, stemmed or custom implants, or bone block arthrodesis.

When the decision to treat osteolysis and cystic lesion has been made, the operation planned depends on the fixation and orientation of the implants. This should be determined preoperatively by serial radiographs and CT scans (>5 mm or 5-degree change in alignment on serial imaging).[9] Removing well-fixed, integrated implants is difficult and removes a substantial amount of bone and is therefore reserved for malorientation that contributes to excessive UHMWPE insert wear. The replacement set should be available at the time of bone grafting because sometimes the radiologic evidence of loosening is lacking and on intraoperative probing, either the tibia or talus is loose. UHMWPE insert exchange is a routine part of the surgical procedure to reduce the source of wear particles. Other causes of excessive wear, such as ankle instability or hindfoot deformity, should be looked for and treated. The revised explanted UHMWPE insert must be examined for excessive wear (**Fig. 2**). This may indicate that one of the previously mentioned problems may need addressing during that surgical episode.

Cystic lesions should be exposed and curetted to bleeding bone substrate. Specimens should be sent for culture and histologic analysis in all cases. Impaction bone grafting with cancellous autograft or lyophilized allograft and demineralized bone matrix of the cyst should be performed (**Fig. 3**). With the older Agility total ankle replacement models, inferior UHMWPE insertion and removal is very difficult with retention of the implant. Techniques to perform this are discussed later.

TALAR SUBSIDENCE

Before the introduction of the Agility LP total ankle replacement system,[6] the original Agility total ankle replacement system's talar component covered only 38% of the cut talar surface. Focal load through the small undersurface led to a high incidence of subsidence into the body of the talus. Together with the subsidence, bone tends to overgrow around the edges of the implant leading to impingement of the medial and lateral gutters and the anterior tibia.

Initially, overgrowth was thought to be an isolated process and attempts to remove the bone surgically gave only temporary improvement in range of motion and

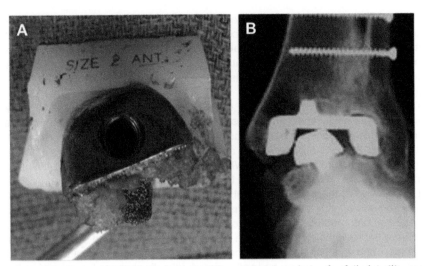

Fig. 2. Intraoperative photograph demonstrating retrieval analysis of a failed Agility total ankle replacement with the talus and polyethylene insert revealing excessive wear (*A*) caused by hindfoot malalignment and medial ankle instability as demonstrated on the anteroposterior radiograph (*B*) of the same patient before revision.

symptoms. It is now known that the two processes are linked and simple bone removal is not a definitive solution. Subsidence has been less of a problem since the introduction of the Agility LP total ankle replacement design in 2006.[6,7] This increased the cut talar surface coverage to 85% by adding medial and lateral flares to the base of the implant.[6] This has also provided a valuable option for reconstruction in certain talar revision cases (**Fig. 4**).

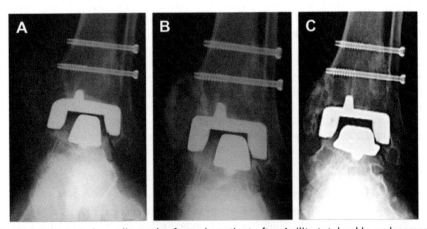

Fig. 3. Anteroposterior radiograph of a male patient after Agility total ankle replacement presenting with medial malleolar pain and swelling 3-years postoperative. (*A*) The polyethylene was exchanged and the talar component changed to the Agility LP version because it was loose at the time of surgery. Two follow-up radiographs early (*B*) and long-term (*C*) postrevision demonstrating progressive maturation and incorporation. The tibia remained well fixed.

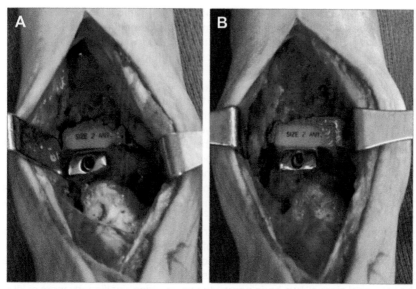

Fig. 4. Intraoperative photograph demonstrating talar subsidence and bone overgrowth, before (*A*) and after (*B*) debridement of the gutters. As noted in the text, this is not an adequate method of treating bone overgrowth because subsidence invariably accompanies this type of bone formation.

Patients with talar subsidence present with decreasing range of motion and increasing mechanical pain caused by the impingement. Radiographs, particularly the weightbearing lateral ankle view, illustrate the subsidence. This can be measured by the distance from the inferior part of the prosthesis to the lateral process of the talus (**Fig. 5**).

Serial radiographs are useful to document progression. Bone overgrowth of the perimeter is often a feature. CT scanning is essential to evaluate the integrity of the talus, the degree of subsidence, and the proximity of the implant to the subtalar joint.

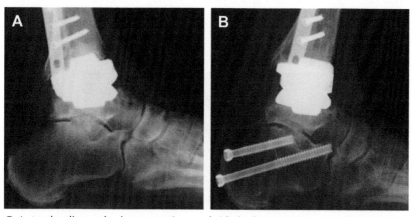

Fig. 5. Lateral radiographs demonstrating a subsided talar component, grade 2 (*A*) that was revised to an Agility LP talus with calcaneus osteotomy and polyethylene exchange (*B*).

(Ellington and Myerson, personal communication, 2012) provided a grading system from 1 to 3. Grade 3 is where the talus has migrated onto or through the subtalar joint. In grade 2, the prosthesis has not disturbed the subtalar joint but has subsided into the talar body. In grade 1, there is minimal subsidence (**Fig. 6**). This has been shown to correlate with outcome after revision.[18]

In most cases, talar subsidence is isolated with a well-fixed and aligned tibial component. In the situations where both the tibia and talus are loose or have subsided, a complete revision of both needs to be done but this is not usual nowadays because the tibial components that were well-fixed years ago tend to remain so. If loose, revision to a different prosthesis system or another Agility LP total ankle replacement talus and tibia is possible.[6] To remove a well-fixed and aligned tibial component seems a pity considering the difficulty and resulting bone loss. For this reason the authors try and retain the tibial component if possible. For the talus, the surgical options are to revise with an Agility total ankle replacement standard revision or LP talus or, alternatively, to use a custom stemmed implant.[2,19,20] The decision is based on the degree of subsidence and proximity to the subtalar joint, the presence of osteopenia, cysts, and evidence of subtalar arthritis. Cases of severe subsidence (late grade 2 and 3) or predicted inability of the talus to support a revision standard talus component should receive a stemmed custom prosthesis (**Fig. 7**).[2,19,20]

The calcaneal stem allows bone ongrowth and provides significantly more axial and rotational stability. The subtalar joint has to be prepared separately through a sinus tarsi incision as the stem crosses it and forms part of the arthrodesis. Screw augmentation across the joint aids stability of the arthrodesis. The implantation requires careful planning with CT scans and radiographs because stem angles and talar body sizes have to be determined beforehand. Templates are provided to confirm the correct size and orientation before final manufacturing. Custom revision instrumentation, reamers, and trial implants are provided in the set.[2]

A standard Agility revision talus is applicable in grade 1 and early grade 2 subsidence with good bone stock. The wider Agility LP talus covers more of the surface and provided the bone quality is adequate, incorporates well with little subsequent subsidence.[6]

The intraoperative difficulties encountered are technical. The older tibial components required insertion or removal of the UHMWPE insert on the inferior surface of the tibial component, which is difficult with a retained talus. The UHMWPE insert also had full-length medial and lateral column locking mechanisms making removal extremely difficult (**Fig. 8**).

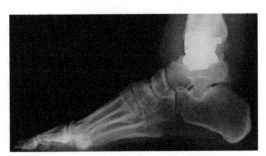

Fig. 6. Lateral radiograph demonstrating grade 2 talar subluxation with well-fixed tibial component.

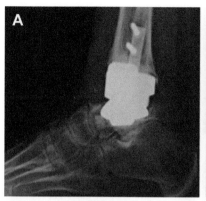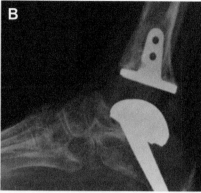

Fig. 7. Lateral radiograph demonstrating grade 3 talar subsidence with a loose tibial component. (*A*) Revision of the talar component requires a custom stemmed prosthesis and subtalar arthrodesis. (*B*) The tibia was also revised using the Salto Talaris prosthesis. Note the improved alignment of the tibial component and the secure fixation of the talar component. The orientation of the talar component is slightly extended, but has not restricted range of motion. This customized long stem device is no longer made available by DePuy Orthopedics.

Newer-generation tibial components have a front-loading mechanism for the UHMWPE insert.[6] Removal of the talus, even if loose, with the UHMWPE insert in place is also very difficult because of the subsidence and subsequent contraction of the joint space. Occasionally, a loose talus can be levered out with distraction of the joint and then the UHMWPE inserts columns pried open with the use of an osteotome or even cut out with a reciprocal saw (**Fig. 9**). When it is impossible to remove the talus first, the columns of the UHMWPE insert locking mechanism can be broken by forcefully inserting an osteotome into the small space between the implant and the polyethylene and then removing the talus secondarily. After preparation of the talar

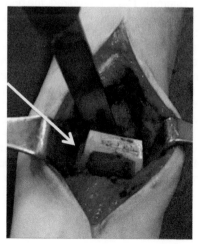

Fig. 8. Intraoperative photograph showing difficulty removing the polyethylene and the full-length column (*arrow*).

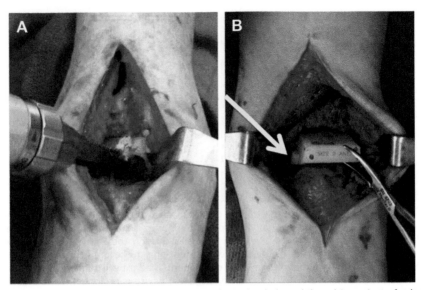

Fig. 9. Use of a reciprocating saw to remove the polyethylene (*A*) and insertion of a half-column polyethylene component (*arrow*) (*B*). The half-column polyethylene is a standard component for this system and is not a customized device. With the half-column, it is slightly (but not always completely) easier to insert by sliding the polyethylene insert in from anterior rather than inferior, which is invariably blocked by the position of the talus and soft tissue contracture.

surface, eliminating defects and grafting cysts, the revision Agility LP talus is impacted. This leaves another problem: how to get the new UHMWPE insert into the tibial component? This is very difficult even with the new half-length column UHMWPE inserts. If it is impossible to get it in with distraction and plantar flexion, complete removal of the columns with an oscillating saw allows the polyethylene to slide in from anterior but it then does not lock into the base plate.

In cases where a custom stemmed talus is required, the previously mentioned problems with UHMWPE insert removal and insertion are similar but accurate insertion of the talus is also difficult. Even when the UHMWPE is removed, to get the correct trajectory of the guidewire down the calcaneus requires joint distraction and circumferential soft tissue release. The use of distracting devices is very helpful. A guidewire and then sequential reamers are passed retrograde from the talar neck into the calcaneus. Trial implants are used to determine if adequate reaming and bone resection have been performed and then the definitive custom implant is inserted.[2]

First-generation Agility implants could not mismatch the talar, tibial, and polyethylene sizes.[7] There was also no modularity of the polyethylene thickness.[7] Newer-generation implants allow the insertion of a larger talar component than the tibia to cover more talar surface and a wider range of UHMWPE insert thicknesses exist to balance the soft tissues of the joint.[6] It is important that all the trial implants and a range of definitive implants be available in theater.

TIBIAL SUBSIDENCE

Lucent lines around the tibial implant are very common and described as well-circumscribed, linear, and not exceeding 1.25 mm on fine-cut CT scan or 2 mm on plain radiographs.[15] They appear before 2 years postimplantation, are not progressive, and loosening or implant migration is not a feature. The cause of these lines is not clear but they seem to be benign. Tibial subsidence may be the result of osteolysis and cyst formation, previous revision with excessive bone loss, severe host osteopenia, undersizing of the implant, periprosthetic fracture, and previous infection (**Fig. 10**).

Tibial revision surgery can be challenging because there is often substantial bone loss and the defects can be large and uncontained (**Fig. 11**). The treating surgeon, after reviewing CT scans, needs to decide if the distal tibia will support a conventional nonstemmed implant or if there is a need for stemmed implant.[2]

Generally, if 50% of the distal tibial plafond remains intact with good bone quality, a conventional implant will be supported after impaction bone grafting of the metaphyseal defect.[2] The joint line level will have to be recreated with a thicker UHMWPE insert (**Fig. 12**).

A custom implant with a large peg or keel that bypasses the defect into better proximal bone should be considered when severe bone loss is present. This provides additional stability to resist subsidence as graft incorporates and ongrowth occurs. They come in various sizes and some have proximal holes for screw locking options, further stabilizing the construct. One disadvantage is the large cortical window necessary for implantation of these prostheses, which often require internal fixation themselves. Learning from revision hip replacement surgery, an intramedullary press fit long stem (INBONE total ankle replacement system; Wright Medical, Inc, Arlington, TN) is designed for massive defects with no metaphyseal support. One of the distinct advantages with this particular total ankle replacement system is that a cortical window is not necessary because the implant is inserted modularly retrograde through the tibial base. This is an exciting concept but there is little evidence to support or refute the implant at this time.

It should be clear that bone grafting is essential in revision cases. Cortical defects with large communicating metaphyseal defects are uncontained and require structural grafting with fresh frozen allograft.[19] Metaphyseal defects have to be impaction bone grafted. Small defects are amenable to cancellous autograft from the iliac crest or proximal tibia but larger defects require a combination of the above and cancellous allograft mixed with demineralized bone matrix. Impaction of the graft to form a stable level distal tibia is important for stability and incorporation. A broad flat osteotome the size of the distal tibia inserted from anterior to posterior is a good tool to force bone graft into the tibial defects, creating a flat surface for the implant.

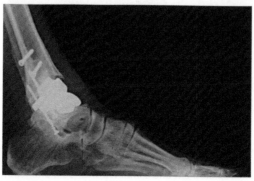

Fig. 10. Lateral radiograph demonstrating significant tibial subsidence and extension.

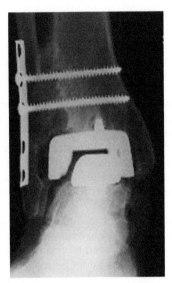

Fig. 11. Anteroposterior radiograph demonstrating significant cyst formation medially and laterally with metaphyseal lucency. A CT scan should be obtained to plan the revision surgery.

Trabecular metal technology (Zimmer, Inc, Warsaw, IN) has exceptional bone ongrowth potential and is used extensively in hip and knee revision arthroplasty. It has also been used for ankle arthrodesis.[21] One of the major benefits is the modularity and variety of sizes and shapes of the augments. Custom shaping is also practiced in the hip and knee and may become possible in the distal tibia to fill large irregular defects. One serious disadvantage is the major procedure required to remove the metal after bone ongrowth has occurred in cases with active infection.

In certain exceptional circumstances, polymethylmethacrylate cement placed around the tibial implant may be used to provide immediate stability where the distal

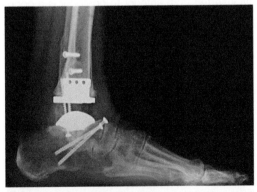

Fig. 12. Lateral radiograph of the same patient shown in **Fig. 10** demonstrating tibial subsidence treated with impaction cancellous bone grafting and revision with a conventional Salto Talaris total ankle replacement and combined with a simultaneously performed subtalar arthrodesis.

tibia is grossly deficient in a patient who requires early weightbearing. Very low demand patients with rheumatoid arthritis or geriatric patients undergoing revision surgery who cannot tolerate a prolonged period of immobilization fall into this small category. This is not a biologic fixation and likely to fail catastrophically at the cement bone interface in active patients.

SUBSIDENCE OF THE TIBIA AND TALUS

When the tibial and talar components have subsided requiring revision, each side of the joint has to be treated separately on its own merits. A good revision system is necessary to address both problems. This may require compatible custom implants.

ASEPTIC LOOSENING

After it was established that polymethylmethacrylate cemented total ankle replacements had poor outcomes because of loosening at the bone-cement interface, a biologic fixation of the implant to host bone was necessary. Osseous ongrowth is enhanced by implant materials and designs. This is enhanced by grit-blasting, pitting, and hydroxyapatite coating of the titanium implant.[1,2,5] Osseous ongrowth only occurs if there is no micromotion at the implant-bone interface after implantation. Greater than 100 μm of motion leads to fibrous ingrowth and a nonbiologic fixation. This makes surgical technique and press-fit fixation important during the primary procedure.

Sometimes, in total ankle replacement, it may be difficult to distinguish aseptic loosening from an implant that did not undergo bony ongrowth after the primary procedure. The cause of the two scenarios is different but the surgical options are similar. Aseptic loosening is a failure of the bone-implant interface, usually caused by loss of bone and cyst formation. Wear particle generation and dispersion through the effective joint space and between the bone and implant leads to osteolysis. This has been discussed previously.

FRACTURES

Malleolar fractures are fairly common after total ankle replacement. The Agility total ankle replacement prosthesis requires a press-fit between the lateral and medial malleoli and a syndesmotic arthrodesis for lateral stability. The tibial cut is aggressive in the transverse plain and predisposes to malleolar fracture. These fractures can occur during the primary surgery, later during ambulation, or after subsidence of the tibial or talar components (**Fig. 13**).

Intraoperative fractures result from very medial and proximal vertical tibial cuts and if a very posterior fibula is not recognized while making the transverse tibial cut posteriorly. Osteopenic bone is predisposed to fracture but can be prevented by conservative cuts and placement of Kirschner wires or cannulated screw guidewires through the medial malleolus during tibial preparation. If a fracture is noted intraoperatively, it should be anatomically reduced and fixed with two cannulated screws. Fibula fractures are much less common. The Agility total ankle replacement system requires fixation and arthrodesis of the syndesmosis and some surgeons, including the senior author, use screws and a plate to provide fixation.[22] If a fracture is identified, this should be reduced and included in the construct.

Fractures of the medial malleolus need reduction and fixation. Occasionally, they may be minimally displaced or only a stress fracture and difficult to see on plain radiographs. CT scanning in this circumstance is helpful for two reasons: it can identify occult fractures, and it can exclude the presence of a cyst. The cause includes medial

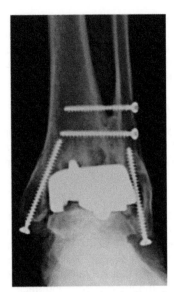

Fig. 13. This subsiding tibia had caused a medial and a lateral malleolar fracture, fixed with screws as demonstrated on the anteroposterior radiograph. This implant needs revision.

malleolar cysts, component varus or valgus malalignment, hindfoot malalignment, ligament instability, and tibial subsidence. As the tibia subsides, the anteromedial talus impinges on the medial malleolus repetitively causing either a stress fracture or an acute fracture. Clinically the patients have local malleolar pain, swelling, and deformity if displaced.

JOINT-SACRIFICING SALVAGE

There are situations when reconstruction with a revision total ankle replacement is not feasible. The decision to proceed to an arthrodesis is sometimes easy to make because of gross bone loss and implant failure but sometimes the decision is more difficult when custom implants can possibly salvage the joint but the chance of biologic fixation and function is questionable (**Fig. 14**). The patient needs to be involved in the decision-making process after all the risks and benefits have been discussed.

Many failed total ankle replacements requiring salvage have significant bone defects making arthrodesis complicated. Large structural bone graft is necessary and the subtalar joint often needs to be included in the arthrodesis to obtain adequate fixation. Fusion rates and graft incorporation are inferior to primary arthrodesis and the complication rate is higher (**Fig. 15**). Surgery is performed through a scarred soft tissue envelope and the bone perfusion is compromised after the peri-implant osteolysis.

When enough talar and distal tibial bone remains, an in situ tibiotalar fusion is possible. The senior author prefers using an anterior arthrodesis plate because there is already a large anterior incision for implant removal and the joint is well visualized. If significant defects exist, structural bone graft is necessary to bridge the tibiotalar gap and obtain anatomic length of the ankle and hindfoot (**Fig. 16**).

When the subtalar joint is arthritic or the talar bone loss significant and not likely to adequately hold internal fixation, a tibiotalocalcaneal arthrodesis is indicated. Either a retrograde locked compression intramedullary nail with subtalar joint preparation

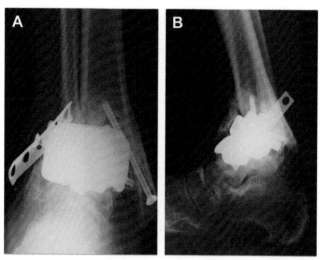

Fig. 14. Anteroposterior (A) and lateral (B) radiographs of a failed Agility total ankle replacement demonstrating obvious loosing and gross failure of tibial and talar components with significant bone loss. Because of the magnitude of tibial component subsidence, revision requires resection of too much of the posterior tibia to create a planar surface for prosthesis support. Joint salvage is not an option in this case because there is too much bone loss and absent fibular support and a tibiotalocalcaneal arthrodesis is necessary.

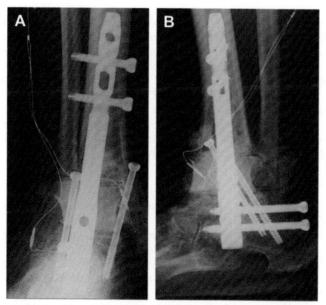

Fig. 15. Anteroposterior (A) and lateral (B) radiographs of the same patient shown in **Fig. 14** after salvage with retrograde locked compression intramedually nail fixation, internal bone growth stimulation, and a bulk bone graft block.

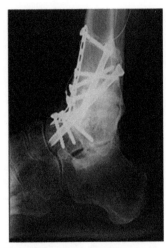

Fig. 16. Lateral radiograph demonstrating ankle fusion with a structural bone block graft and sparing of the subtalar joint because good bone stock was available in the remaining talus.

or an anterior plate with supplementary screw fixation of the subtalar joint provide sufficient internal fixation for compression and fusion. The decision to perform either an isolated tibiotalar arthrodesis or a tibiotalocalcaneal arthrodesis (both with structural grafting) is made according to the amount of talar bone still present and a symptomatic subtalar joint.

SUMMARY

The Agility total ankle replacement system was the most commonly implanted Food and Drug Administration–cleared implant for more than 20 years. Predictably, as time has progressed the need for revision has increased. Predictable modes of failure occur and likewise a step-wise revision process can be tailored to each case and patient-specific needs. The authors present 15 years of primary implantation of the Agility total ankle replacement system and significant experience with revision of this particular total ankle replacement system to optimize patient outcome. The potential need to revise already revised Agility total ankle replacements exists and only surgeons experienced with the particulars of this system and the revision requirements should undertake this complex surgery.

REFERENCES

1. Gougoulias NE, Khanna A, Maffulli N. History and evolution in total ankle arthroplasty. Br Med Bull 2009;89:111–51.
2. Myerson MS, Won HY. Primary and revision total ankle replacement using custom-designed prostheses. Foot Ankle Clin 2008;13:521–38.
3. Labek G, Thaler M, Janda W, et al. Revision rates after total joint replacement: cumulative results from worldwide joint register datasets. J Bone Joint Surg Br 2011;93:293–7.
4. Henricson A, Nilsson JÅ, Carlsson A. 10-year survival of total ankle arthroplasties: a report on 780 cases from the Swedish Ankle Register. Acta Orthop 2011;82: 655–9.

5. de Steiger RN, Hang JR, Miller LN, et al. Five year results of the ASR XL acetabular system and ASR hip resurfacing: an analysis from the Australian Association National Joint Registry. J Bone Joint Surg Am 2011;93:2287–93.
6. Cerrato R, Myerson MS. Total ankle replacement: the Agility LP prosthesis. Foot Ankle Clin 2008;13:485–94.
7. Roukis TS. Incidence of revision after primary implantation of the Agility total ankle replacement system: a systematic review. J Foot Ankle Surg 2012;51: 198–204.
8. Guyer AJ, Richardson EG. Current concepts review: total ankle arthroplasty. Foot Ankle Int 2008;29:256–64.
9. Pyevich MT, Saltzman CL, Callaghan JJ, et al. Total ankle arthroplasty: a unique design. Two to twelve-year follow-up. J Bone Joint Surg Am 1998;80:1410–20.
10. Knecht SI, Estin M, Callaghan JJ, et al. The Agility total ankle arthroplasty. Seven to sixteen-year follow-up. J Bone Joint Surg Am 2004;86:1161–71.
11. Gougoulias N, Khanna A, Maffulli N. How successful are current ankle replacements? A systematic review of the literature. Clin Orthop Relat Res 2010;468: 199–208.
12. Iwakiri K, Minoda Y, Kobayashi A, et al. In vivo comparison of wear particles between highly cross linked polyethylene and conventional polyethylene. J Biomed Mater Res B Appl Biomater 2009;91:799–804.
13. Rodriguez D, Bevernage BD, Maldague P, et al. Medium term follow-up of the AES ankle prosthesis: high rate of asymptomatic osteolysis. Foot Ankle Surg 2010;16:54–60.
14. Vaupel Z, Baker E, Baker KC, et al. Analysis of retrieved agility total ankle arthroplasty systems. Foot Ankle Int 2009;30(9):815–23.
15. Hanna RS, Haddad SL, Lazarus ML. Evaluation of peri-prosthetic lucency after total ankle arthroplasty: helical CT versus conventional radiography. Foot Ankle Int 2007;28:921–6.
16. Paprosky WG, Magnus RE. Principles of bone grafting in revision total hip arthroplasty-acetabular technique. Clin Orthop Relat Res 1994;298:147–55.
17. Bonnin M, Gaudot F, Laurent J-R, et al. The Salto total ankle arthroplasty: survivorship and analysis of failures at 7 to 11-years. Clin Orthop Relat Res 2011;469: 225–36.
18. Ketz J, Myerson M, Sanders R. The salvage of complex hindfoot problems with use of a custom talar total ankle prosthesis. J Bone Joint Surg Am 2012;94(13): 1194–200.
19. Myerson MS. Revision total ankle replacement. In: Myserson MS, editor. Reconstructive foot and ankle surgery: management of complications. 2nd edition. Philadelphia: Elsevier Saunders; 2010. p. 295–316.
20. Ketz J, Myerson MS, Sanders R. The salvage of complex hindfoot problems with use of a custom talar total ankle prosthesis. J Bone Joint Surg Am 2012;94: 1194–200.
21. Henricson A, Rydholm U. Use of a trabecular metal implant in ankle arthrodesis after failed total ankle replacement. Acta Orthop 2010;81:745–7.
22. Jung H-G, Nicholson JJ, Parks B, et al. Radiographic and biomechanical support for fibular plating of the agility total ankle. Clin Orthop Relat Res 2004;424: 118–24.

Revision INBONE Total Ankle Replacement

James K. DeOrio, MD

KEYWORDS

- INBONE • Total ankle replacement • Total ankle arthroplasty • Revision
- Ankle arthritis

KEY POINTS

- The INBONE total ankle replacement is an excellent primary and revision ankle replacement because of its modularity and the ability to make up any tibial bone loss.
- Revision of the INBONE total ankle replacement may be necessary, however, because of poor patient selection, technique error, or infection.
- If it is because of poor patient selection, then other specialty consultations (eg, plastic surgery for free tissue transfer) may be needed to provide patients the best care possible.
- If the ankle needs to be reoperated on because of a technical error, then often that additional surgery can be performed in a second stage.
- Finally, if the ankle needs to be removed (eg, infection), doing so posteriorly and filling the defect with a femoral head and securing it with a retrograde compression locked intramedullary nail can give patients a very functional limb.

INTRODUCTION

Although there are specific components designed for revision hip, knee, and even shoulder replacement, in the United States, no such prosthesis exists for ankle replacement, although custom talar prostheses have been used.[1] Instead, when appropriate, surgeons must rely on primary prostheses and surgical technique to salvage total ankle replacements that have failed. Fortunately, the failure rate is generally low, 5% to 15% at 8 to 12 years.[2] Other studies[3] cite a higher failure rate, increasing the importance of articles like this one. When using off-the-shelf bulk prostheses for revisions, one surgeon reported results as "good" in 83% of revisions accomplished.[4] In my opinion, the INBONE (Wright Medical Technology, Arlington, Tennessee) ankle offers a good primary and revision/replacement ankle. What should be done, however, when the INBONE total ankle replacement fails? This article discusses the reasons for

Dr DeOrio is a consultant for the manufacturer of the INBONE ankle, Wright Medical Technology (Arlington, Tennessee).
Department of Orthopaedic Surgery, Duke University Medical Center, Duke Medical Plaza, 4709 Creekstone Drive Suite 200, Durham, NC 27703, USA
E-mail address: James.deorio@duke.edu

Clin Podiatr Med Surg 30 (2013) 225–236
http://dx.doi.org/10.1016/j.cpm.2012.10.003
0891-8422/13/$ – see front matter © 2013 Elsevier Inc. All rights reserved.

failure of primary and revision INBONE total ankle replacements and how to reconstruct the ankle.

The INBONE total ankle replacement is unique. With the new INBONE II design, the talar component has a V-shaped platform with a matching ultrahigh molecular weight polyethylene (UHMWPE) design firmly attached to the tibial component. A more detailed insertion technique is included in an article by DeOrio.[5] Previously, the INBONE talar component was a saddle-shaped design but the saddle did not have enough medial-to-lateral stability, so the change is a good one. The INBONE total ankle replacement is unique in that it has multiple pieces that are screwed together to create a stem to go up into the tibia. To do so, a 6-mm hole is drilled from the plantar calcaneus up the calcaneus, then the talus, and into the tibia. The medullary portion of the tibia is then reamed out and the tibial components screwed into one another to form the stem. Added to the central stem on the INBONE II talar component are 2 anterior pegs that help control rotation. These are appropriate and the author has moved exclusively to INBONE II for his patients.

The technique for insertion of the tibial stem has required a leg holder with fluoroscopy.[5] There is a new way, however, to insert the INBONE total ankle replacement (Prophecy INBONE Pre-Operative Navigation Alignment Guides, Wright Medical Technology, Arlington, Tennessee). It involves getting a CT scan of a patient's ankle before the surgery and creating plastic molds. These molds are then placed on the bone in the open ankle for exact placement of the cutting jig pins. The plastic molds are removed from the cutting jib pins and the cutting jigs are then placed on the pins that also aid in placement of the long 6-mm drill. The bone can then be cut precisely without need for the leg holder. It is not yet in widespread use, so all the ankles discussed in this article have been done with the leg holder.

REASONS FOR FAILURE

The reasons for failure of the INBONE total ankle replacement include, but are not limited to, poor patient selection. Thus, placing a total ankle in a patient with peripheral vascular disease (can be occult) resulting in a large wound problem necessitates free flap coverage or amputation. At Duke University, the use of a radial forearm flap for severe wound problems has been successful. This has been done without any exchange of the prosthesis. Sending patients for a vascular consultation preoperatively, whenever the dorsalis pedis or posterior tibial pulse is not palpable, may save surgeons and patients a great deal of grief.

The next reason for failure is insertion of a total ankle replacement in patients with avascular necrosis of the talus, most likely from obvious trauma (talar neck fracture) but sometimes without a history of trauma. In **Fig. 1** there is atraumatic avascular necrosis of the talus. The patient has obvious arthritis of the ankle, including the subtalar joint, undergoes an INBONE total ankle replacement; and does well initially. At 6 months, there is some initial collapse of the talar component and 1 year later there is significant painful collapse of the talar component. She subsequently undergoes tibiotalocalcaneal arthrodesis with a retrograde locked compression intramedullary nail and femoral head allograft to fill the void and does well (**Fig. 2**).

I have also seen this phenomenon of talar collapse in all commercially available models of total ankle replacement when too much bone is resected from the talus. Salvage is then virtually impossible. Although the creators of the INBONE total ankle replacement contend that the drill evades the arterial supply of the talus, I believe that in some patients, unique patterning of the talar vascularity makes it susceptible to damage in a low-cut talus. In **Fig. 3**, a 73-year-old man undergoes an INBONE total

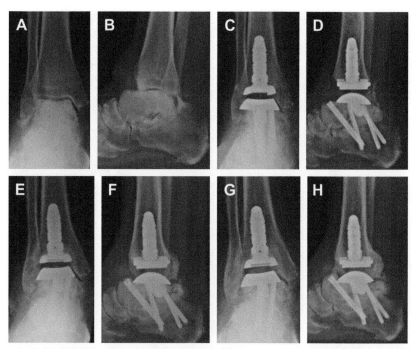

Fig. 1. Increased sclerosis can be appreciated on the anteroposterior radiograph (*A*) of a 68-year-old female patient with talar avascular necrosis possibly secondary to smoking tobacco. On the lateral view (*B*), the subtalar joint is significantly narrowed with shrinkage of the talus. Anteroposterior (*C*) and lateral (*D*) radiographs at 6 weeks demonstrate good alignment and no subsidence. Anteroposterior radiograph (*E*) at 6 months looks good; however, the lateral view (*F*) demonstrates early evidence of subsidence. At 1 year, there is progressive subsidence appreciated on the anteroposterior (*G*) and lateral (*H*) radiographs.

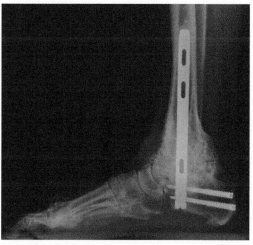

Fig. 2. The same patient demonstrated in **Fig. 1** had continued pain and was treated with a tibiotalocalcaneal arthrodesis and at 1 year postoperative the patient is doing great and playing golf 4 times a week. Note that there is good alignment and a femoral head allograft was used from a posterior approach to fill in the defect left after the prosthesis had been removed.

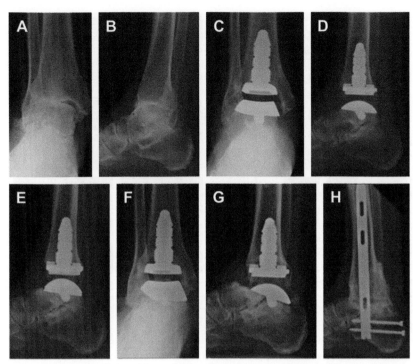

Fig. 3. Anteroposterior (*A*) and lateral (*B*) radiographs of a 73-year-old man with a 2-year history of ankle pain. Postoperative anteroposterior radiograph with no irregularities appreciated (*C*). The lateral view demonstrates a slight tapered talar cut taking more bone posteriorly than anteriorly (*D*). A lateral radiograph at 6 months demonstrates moderate posterior collapse with mild pain (*E*). Anteroposterior (*F*) and lateral (*G*) radiographs at 21 months demonstrate complete posterior collapse but only moderate pain. Revision with a tibiotalocalcaneal arthrodesis using a retrograde compression locked intramedullary nail and femoral head allograft demonstrating primary osseous integration (*H*). The patient is doing well.

ankle replacement. There was perhaps slightly more bone taken on the talus posteriorly than is appropriate and the patient subsequently undergoes collapse of the talus under the talar component. He, too, is ultimately provided a tibiotalocalcaneal arthrodesis with a retrograde locked compression intramedullary nail and femoral head allograft that enables him to keep up his sporting activities. Although there are reports in the literature of using so-called metal reinforced cement augmentation to support the body weight, I have not had success with this technique when the bone is avascular.[6] Hence, I prefer to perform a tibiotalocalcaneal arthrodesis rather than attempt revision total ankle replacement in this setting.

When avascular necrosis of the talus is suspected, obtain an MRI preoperatively and assess the remaining blood supply to the talus. In my practice, if there is less than 75% of the talus with good blood supply remaining and in contact with the talar component after talar resection, then there is increased risk of collapse and I believe the patient is better served with an arthrodesis as the index surgery rather than after failure of a total ankle replacement.

Other patients in whom increased risk is assumed by patients and surgeons when performing a total ankle replacement include patients with peripheral sensory and/or motor neuropathy, patients with clubfoot deformity because the fibula lies immediately posterior to the talus, patients whose lifestyle is physically aggressive, patients less than 40 years old, and patients with insulin therapy for diabetes mellitus. Avoiding total ankle replacement in these patients increases overall rates of success and decreases the need to perform revision total ankle replacement. Note that weight is not included because the weight issue has been shown to be less of a problem than originally believed.[7] At the same time, a high body mass index and obesity have not been able to be lowered by providing patients with a pain-free ankle replacement.[8] The patient shown in **Fig. 4** is an extremely active patient, not obese. The patient did well postoperatively and returned to all his former activities, including carrying a canoe down to the river as a whitewater raft instructor. The goal in patients like this is difficult and it is to convince those with no pain that they must moderate their activities. This patient, at 3 years postoperative, underwent revision UHMWPE exchange with clean out of his tibial cyst and insertion of calcium phosphate (**Fig. 5**). If he continues to be symptomatic, he will need a complete INBONE II revision ankle replacement.

The next groups of patients, who are infrequent, are those posttraumatic patients with a nonunion of the tibia. In these cases, the INBONE is particularly susceptible to a fatigue fracture because of its small-diameter, 6-mm threaded stem connectors. Hence, it is not the actual 12-mm to 18-mm stem pieces that take the stress but rather their threaded connectors that are only 6 mm in diameter. So too, the Morse taper

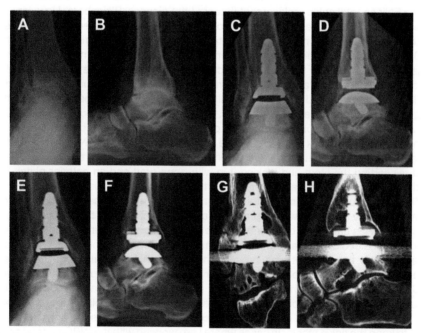

Fig. 4. Anteroposterior (*A*) and lateral (*B*) radiographs from a 62-year-old man with arthritis from multiple sprains. Note that the subtalar joint is free of disease. Anteroposterior (*C*) and lateral (*D*) radiographs at 1 year postoperative look good. Anteroposterior (*E*) and lateral (*F*) radiographs at 3 years postoperative demonstrate osteolysis about the tibial stem. Frontal (*G*) and sagittal (*H*) CT scan images demonstrate that the osteolysis and cystic changes are larger than appreciated on the plain film radiographs.

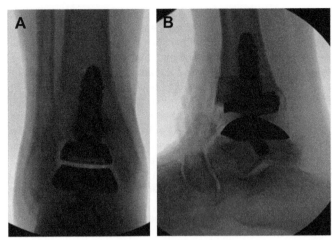

Fig. 5. Anteroposterior (*A*) and lateral (*B*) intraoperative image intensification views after UHMWPE insert exchange and débridement of the osteolytic cysts, followed by insertion of calcium phosphate into the tibial cyst.

connector between the tibial base plate and the base stem is at risk for failure. Two such cases are discussed. **Fig. 6** shows a case of using the INBONE as a revision of the Eclipse total ankle replacement (Integra LifeSciences, Plainsboro, New Jersey). The original surgeon used a medial approach for the Eclipse total ankle replacement that went on to nonunion. The Eclipse total ankle replacement was removed and the INBONE inserted, but, because the patient had diabetes mellitus, minimal dissection was performed medially to limit vascular compromise. The defective medial malleolus was bone grafted and stabilized with 2 compression screws. Unfortunately, the medial malleolar osteotomy did not heal and, ultimately, the threaded post coming off the base stem piece fatigued and fractured. The patient was returned to surgery, iliac crest autograft and a robust plate were placed medially, and the patient kept strict non–weight bearing. Six weeks later, the patient underwent INBONE revision of the tibial piece only by lifting off a 2-cm window of bone, removing the broken stem, and reinserting the stem and locking it in with bone graft and an anterior plate. The patient has done well to date and returned to all normal activity.

The second patient is similar to the patient in **Fig. 6** and had severe trauma to his lower extremity (**Fig. 7**). It was appreciated at the time of surgery that the medial split in the tibia was unhealed, but it was believed that bone grafting and minimal fixation would suffice. It did not heal and the Morse taper stem coming off the base plate fractured. By the time patient was revised, the nonunion had healed but the patient needed revision because of the fractured implant. The fractured parts were removed and a new INBONE total ankle replacement inserted. A word of caution: just because a surgeon is able to get a prosthesis removed and a new one in place does not mean the surgeon will be able to establish the necessary tension across the polytalar interface to keep the ankle stable. In cases where I am working with the INBONE total ankle replacement, I have been able to bring the tibial component down to the talus by inserting a tricortical femoral head allograft beneath the end of the tibia and relying on the intraosseous stem for stability on the tibial side.

The next major category of need for revision total ankle replacement is technical errors. Errors and the technique of revision are discussed. Placement of the ankle in

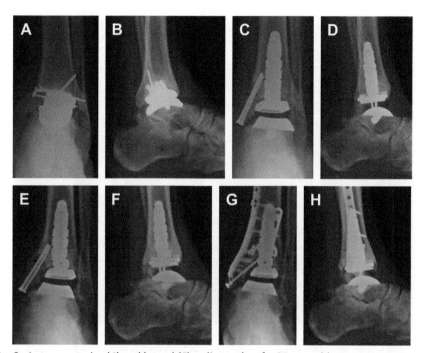

Fig. 6. Anteroposterior (*A*) and lateral (*B*) radiographs of a 67-year-old man status posttraumatic ankle injury in 1954 treated with an Eclipse total ankle replacement in 2007. He has an ankle arthrodesis on the contralateral side. Anteroposterior (*C*) and lateral (*D*) radiographs 3 months' status post–INBONE total ankle replacement with 2-screw fixation and bone grafting of the medial malleolar nonunion Anteroposterior (*E*) and lateral (*F*) radiographs demonstrating obvious nonunion of the medial malleolus with fractured hardware and varus drift of the foot. Anteroposterior (*G*) and lateral (*H*) radiographs demonstrating repair of the nonunion with robust medial plate and screw construct with autogenous iliac crest bone grafting of the nonunion site shown at 2 years postoperative. The broken INBONE prosthesis between distal segments 1 and 2 was also replaced.

greater than 10° of varus or valgus is problematic. Avoiding this problem with liberal use of intraoperative image intensification is advised. If somehow it occurs, at 6 months postoperative for a varus deformity, I do a direct approach opening wedge osteotomy of the medial tibia, using a robust plate on the tibia and doing a separate osteotomy of the fibula at the level of the ankle and plating it with a thinner fibular plate commonly used for ankle fractures. The other choice is a closing wedge resection from the lateral fibula and tibia. This too can be used with success; however, because many of these legs are short, my preference is for the opening wedge. For the valgus deformity, a wedge of bone can be resected from the medial tibia, 4 cm from the tip of the medial malleolus, and plated, or an opening wedge can be done laterally, plating both bones and adding bone graft. Although theoretically the stem blocks the screw placement, in actuality. The screws can be placed anteriorly or posteriorly to the stem. Fortunately, altering the varus or valgus to the degree that requires an osteotomy is seldom required.

I almost never do a varus ankle without a medial deltoid release.[8] **Fig. 8** demonstrates a case in which the medial release was not enough to bring the ankle in to a neutral

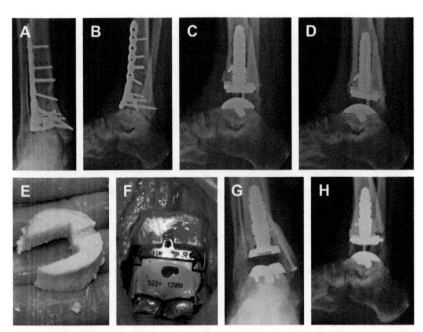

Fig. 7. Anteroposterior (*A*) and lateral (*B*) radiographs of a 68-year-old man who fell at home and underwent open reduction with internal fixation 1 year prior to his INBONE ankle replacement. Lateral radiograph at 6 months postoperatively (*C*) looks good; however, at 1 year postoperative (*D*) notice that the tibial tray is no longer perpendicular to the base stem and the Morse taper has fractured. Intraoperative photograph of the hand-tailored tricortical femoral head allograft (*E*) that is placed between the native distal tibia and INBONE total ankle replacement tibial tray (*F*) in addition to use of revision UHMWPE insert to re-establish proper tension in the ankle. Anteroposterior (*G*) and lateral (*H*) radiographs demonstrating restoration of length and alignment.

position. Thus, I returned the patient to outpatient surgery where I did an opening wedge osteotomy[9,10] of the medial malleolus.

Obtaining balance in a total ankle replacement is critical. For a varus ankle, it has to be determined whether to do a medial slide or a medial malleolar osteotomy. In the radiographs in **Fig. 8**, perhaps the INBONE II would have given enough medial-to-lateral stability, but a medial slide in the face of this severe 24° varus deformity with a shortened protruding medial malleolus deformity ("horizontal" medial malleolus) was ultimately not enough with the original INBONE total ankle replacement. In a second operation, however, I was able to take down the prominence of the medial malleolus by doing a medial malleolar open wedged osteotomy filled with iliac crest bone graft and covered by a plate along with a Bröstrom lateral ankle ligament reconstruction. When making these incisions so close to one another, there is nothing wrong with staging the operations. The key is to avoid the second operation by getting the balance right during the index surgery. It is possible that the INBONE II, with its greater protection against medial and lateral instability, would have prevented such an imbalance.

Fracture of the malleolus intraoperatively is typically not a problem and is fixed at that time with a plate and/or screws. Usually, two 4-mm intramedullary screws are all that is needed. When it is noticed or occurs postoperatively, however, it can either be watched

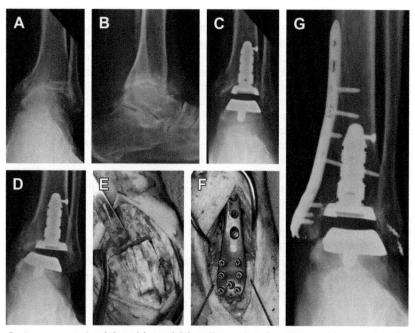

Fig. 8. Anteroposterior (*A*) and lateral (*B*) radiographs of a 60-year-old man with chronic ankle instability and pain with 24° varus deformity. Anteroposterior radiograph at 6 weeks postoperative (*C*) and 6 months postoperative (*D*) demonstrating progressive medial subluxation of the foot. Intraoperative photograph demonstrating the medial malleolar osteotomy with distal translation (*E*) stabilized with a robust plate and screw construct (*F*). Anteroposterior radiograph at 6 months postoperative demonstrating restoration of proper ankle alignment after lateral ankle stabilization and distal translation medial malleolar osteotomy (*G*).

in a cast or taken to surgery, where a screw is placed as it would have been if observed intraoperatively. Putting in a prophylactic cannulated screw in each of the malleoli is a common technique to avoid fracture in cases where a surgeon and assistants are retracting as much soft tissue as possible to gain access to the ankle.[11]

A frequent complaint after implantation of the INBONE total ankle replacement is pain in the medial and/or lateral gutters. The problem is believed to be impingement between the talar component and the adjacent malleolar bone. Many times it is mild and by 1 year is largely resolved. At other times, however, despite best efforts at surgery, patients continue to complain of pain. The choice at this point is to do an open arthrotomy and trim down the malleolus with a fine reciprocal saw to relieve the impingement. Because the talar component would have ingrown by this time, the other choice of trying to reduce it in size is deemed more difficult because of the inevitable loss of talar bone with downsizing of the talar component. Trimming the malleoli may even be done arthroscopically.[12] The latter is made easier using a cautery wand to eliminate some of the capsule to visualize the bone, then trimming the bone away with a bur.

Inadequate dorsiflexion is a problem when I do not have a low enough threshold to do either a triple hemisection lengthening of the Achilles tendon intraoperatively or a gastrocnemius recession. My preference is for the gastrocnemius recession done from the posterior medial side through a 3-cm incision. This is a simple procedure done at the time of the index surgery. I have found it difficult, however, to gain much dorsiflexion with a gastrocnemius slide post–total ankle replacement and am thus prepared to do both in a revision case. Additionally, if a leg holder is used, the foot must be brought to 90°; otherwise, the leg holder will not accept it. In these cases, the Achilles must be lengthened before opening the ankle if using the leg holder.

Another cause for a revision total ankle replacement, and not uncommon, is UHMWPE insert revision. Eventually all UHMWPE inserts wear out. If a prosthesis is imbalanced or a patient is active, this occurs sooner rather than later. In this instance, the gutters are cleaned out and an osteotome is used and the UHMWPE insert simply pried out. Sometimes, to loosen the UHMWPE insert, its attachment on the tibial side is drilled out on both sides with a 3.5-mm drill.

Occasionally, the bone does not grow onto the prosthesis. In these instances, the ankle may be revised after 6 months and the original prosthesis reinserted on fresh cuts or a revision prosthesis inserted (described later). In these cases, it must be ensured that patients are not infected.

The final need for revision to be covered in this article is infection. It must be kept in mind that no matter how perfectly the ankle replacement is performed, an infection destroys the finest piece of work. To prevent infection, everyone must be vigilant. Especially while the image intensification C-arm is rotated beneath the table, everyone must be careful not to touch it "to adjust the drapes." Besides meticulous operative technique, preoperative antibiotics are given and continued for 24 hours or until discharge the following day. I also use antibiotics in the irrigation because there is evidence to show that antibiotics in direct contact with the tissue are effective in preventing infection.[13] Finally, I find a place for bone graft and mix a little vancomycin in it as a final protective barrier toward infection.[14] There is evidence to show that antibiotics can be effective if joined with other products, such as polymethylmethacrylate cement, to sterilize the wound. The formula I use is 1.2 g of vancomycin per 80-g of bone graft. Thus, for most patients, it is no more than one-quarter teaspoon vancomycin added to the bone graft.

If patients present after 3 months with an acute infection (less than 2 weeks of symptoms), and the surgeon is worried that that the prosthesis is ingrown and too much bone will be lost with prosthesis removal, the surgeon can do an open arthrotomy with débridement, polyethylene removal and polymethylmethacrylate antibiotic loaded bone cement spacer placement. After 6 weeks of parenteral antibiotics, remove the cement spacer and insert a new UHMWPE insert. If that fails, then the prosthesis needs to be removed and either the parenteral antibiotics repeated going on to total ankle replacement revision, if there is enough bone; or a tibiotalocalcaneal arthrodesis is done if there is evidence of involvement of the subtalar joint; or just an ankle arthrodesis if there is no evidence of involvement of the subtalar joint.

Patients are placed in a well-padded cast at the end of the surgery. This is left on for 3 weeks and the patients are instructed to be non–weight bearing. That cast is removed at 3 weeks and a protective boot placed on the patient unless an additional procedure was done that requires further cast immobilization. All patients are fully weight bearing at 6 weeks.

In an acute infection (less than 3 months), there has not been osseous ingrowth. The prosthesis is removed, a polymethylmethacrylate antibiotic loaded cement spacer placed, the bacteria identified with deep culture procurement, and the patient placed on 6 weeks of parenteral antibiotics. The antibiotics are discontinued, the ankle aspirated, and, if negative, another INBONE total ankle replacement can be placed. In **Fig. 9**, the infection occurred at 10 months, but the patient was immunosuppressed

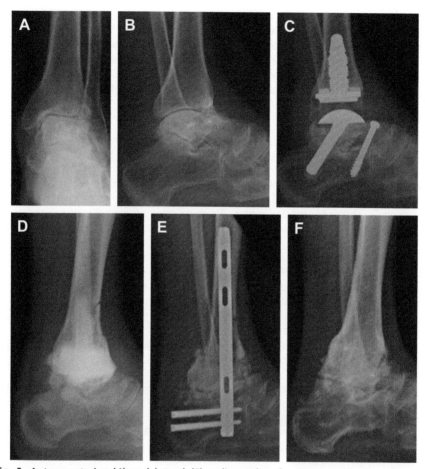

Fig. 9. Anteroposterior (*A*) and lateral (*B*) radiographs of a 63-year-old man with non-Hodgkin lymphoma and ongoing chemotherapy with avascular necrosis of the talus. Lateral radiograph (*C*) at 10 months postoperative demonstrate lucency beneath the posterior aspect of the talar component and along the long stem with a warm and edematous ankle. Lateral radiograph (*D*) after extraction of the INBONE total ankle replacement and placement of an antibiotic-loaded polymethylmethacrylate cement spacer (*D*). Lateral radiograph demonstrating retrograde compression locked intramedullary nail fixation with femoral allograft for a salvage tibiotalocalcaneal arthrodesis 8 weeks later (*E*). Lateral radiograph after removal of the internal fixation due to pain at the proximal aspect of the nail (*F*). Note the likely nonunion of the subtalar joint; however, the patient is doing well.

from chemotherapy and had avascular necrosis of the talus; thus, a tibiotalocalcaneal arthrodesis was performed. Almost 2 years postoperative, the patient complained of pain around the proximal aspect of the nail and thus it was removed.

SUMMARY

Although the INBONE total ankle replacement may be used as a replacement of a failed ankle, it may be used as a primary ankle as well. Not infrequently, the cases I am dealing with often have a severe deformity or significant loss of bone. Those are the kinds of cases that have a higher percentage of reoperation than cases of total ankle replacements in patients without deformity or bone loss. Therefore, comparison rates between ankles have to take that into consideration. Nonetheless, avoidance of some of the problems (discussed previously) will provide patients a good chance of having a solid ankle replacement that can serve them well. Current data collection at Duke University on all its total ankle replacements will hopefully bear this out.

REFERENCES

1. Ketz J, Myerson M, Sanders R. The salvage of complex hindfoot problems with use of a custom talar total ankle prosthesis. J Bone Joint Surg Am 2012;94(13): 1194–2000.
2. Easley M, Adams B, Hembree CW, et al. Results of total ankle arthroplasty. J Bone Joint Surg Am 2011;93(15):1455–60.
3. Labek G, Thaler M, Janda W, et al. Revision rates after total joint replacement: cumulative results from worldwide joint register datasets. J Bone Joint Surg Br 2011;93(3):293–7.
4. Hintermann B, Brag A, Knapp M. Revision arthroplasty of the ankle joint. Orthopade 2011;40(11):1000–7.
5. DeOrio JK. INBONE total ankle replacement: current status. American Academy of Orthopaedic Surgeons Web site: Orthopaedic Knowledge Orthopaedics Online 2011;9(11). Available at: http://orthoportal.org/oko/article.aspx?article=OKO_FOO040#abstract. Accessed November 1, 2011.
6. Schuberth JM, Christensen JC, Rialson JA. Metal-reinforced cement augmentation for complex talar subsidence in failed total ankle arthroplasty. J Foot Ankle Surg 2011;50(6):766–72.
7. Barg A, Knupp M, Anderson AE, et al. Total ankle replacement in obese patients: component stability, weight change, and functional outcome in 118 consecutive patients. Foot Ankle Int 2011;32(10):925–32.
8. Penner MJ, Pakzad H, Younger A, et al. Mean BMI of overweight and obese patients does not decrease after successful ankle reconstruction. J Bone Joint Surg Am 2012;94(9):e57.
9. DeOrio, JK. Ed. S Raikin. INBONE Ankle Replacement. Seminars in Arthroplasty 2010;21(4):288–94.
10. DeOrio JK. INBONE Total Ankle Replacement: Supplementary Procedures. American Academy of Orthopaedic Surgeons Web site: Orthopaedic Knowledge Online 2011;9(11). Available at: http://orthoportal.org/oko/article.aspx?article=OKO_FOO040#abstract. Accessed November 1, 2011.
11. Devries JG, Berlet GC, Lee TH, et al. Revision total ankle replacement: an early look at agility to INBONE. Foot Ankle Surg 2011;50(6):766–72.
12. Richardson AF, DeOrio JK, Parekh SG. Arthroscopic debridement: effective treatment for impingement after total ankle arthroplasty. Curr Rev Musculoskelet Med 2012;5:171–5.
13. Tabutin J, D'Ollonne T, Cambas PM. Antibiotic addition to cement— is it beneficial? Hip Int 2012;22(1):9–12.
14. Chaudhary S, Sen RK, Saini UC, et al. Use of gentamicin-loaded collagen sponge in internal fixation of open fractures. Chin J Traumatol 2011;14(4):209–14.

Incidence of Revision After Primary Implantation of the Scandinavian Total Ankle Replacement System

A Systematic Review

Mark A. Prissel, DPM[a], Thomas S. Roukis, DPM, PhD[b],*

KEYWORDS

• Arthroplasty • Mobile bearing • Prosthesis • STAR • Surgery

KEY POINTS

- Advances in technology for total ankle replacement have renewed the popularity of this procedure as an alternative to ankle arthrodesis.
- Limited information exists regarding long-term survivorship of total ankle replacement, including that of the Scandinavian Total Ankle Replacement.
- National joint arthroplasty registry data provide useful information regarding survivorship of total ankle replacement.
- Total ankle replacement is a demanding procedure that can ultimately fail for a variety of reasons and require revision.
- Revision of total ankle replacement includes metallic component exchange, ankle arthrodesis, and major limb amputation; other joint-involving procedures are termed *reoperations* and non–joint-involving surgeries are considered *additional procedures*.
- Because incidence of failure of total ankle replacement is significant, thorough evaluation of the ankle abnormalities and consideration of revision options are paramount for ultimate total ankle replacement system selection.

INTRODUCTION

Total ankle replacement initially came into favor in the 1970s, with great potential as an alternative to ankle arthrodesis for treatment of advanced ankle arthritis.

Financial Disclosure: None reported.
Conflict of Interest: None reported.
[a] Department of Medical Education, Gundersen Lutheran Medical Foundation, Mail Stop C03-006A, 1836 South Avenue, La Crosse, WI 54601, USA; [b] Department of Orthopaedics, Podiatry and Sports Medicine, Gundersen Lutheran Healthcare System, 2nd Floor Founders Building, Mail Stop FB2-009, 1900 South Avenue, La Crosse, WI 54601, USA
* Corresponding author.
E-mail addresses: tsroukis@gundluth.org; tsrdpm@aol.com

First-generation implants, however, were highly constrained, in retrospect were obviously flawed, and resulted in an unacceptably high incidence of failure, frequently resulting in attempted revision, including component exchange, conversion to arthrodesis, or amputation.[1–5] Current-generation implants, compared with those available decades ago, show promise with greatly improved materials, more precise surgical technique, and increased focus on maintaining the normal anatomy and function of the ankle joint. Mobile-bearing technology has allowed for increased implant conformity, with restriction of implant constraint that theoretically reduces wear and loosening.[6,7] Nevertheless, even with advancements in technology and implant engineering, incidence of implant failure remains a problem still requiring attempted revision.

One current implant is the Scandinavian Total Ankle Replacement (STAR) system, which was invented by Hakon Kofoed, MD and Waldemar Link GmbH & Co. (Hamburg, Germany) in 1978 as an anatomic nonconstrained resurfacing prosthesis. It was first used clinically in 1981, and until 1985 was implanted as a 2-piece design that required cement augmentation. In 1985 it was modified to a 3-piece implant with cobalt chrome tibial and talar components and an ultra-high-molecular-weight polyethylene (UHMWPE) mobile bearing that articulated with both the tibial component and talar component but still required cement augmentation. STAR implant design was further modified in 1990, when it was converted to a cementless double-coated version that included a titanium plasma spray and a 100-μm hydroxyapatite coating on both metallic components. Since 1990, the STAR has been used in its current form, with only minor modifications to the porous coating. The double coating was changed to only a single coating of porous titanium in 1999 with the addition of deposited calcium phosphate. In 2000, metallic radiopaque markers were added to the UHMWPE mobile bearing.[2,3,8–11]

Initial U.S. Food and Drug Administration (FDA) premarket approval for use in the United States was filed on March 24, 2006, with initial approval for general use in April 2007 and ultimate FDA approval on May 27, 2009.[12] Before institution within the United States market, the STAR was available and used across Europe and much of the world. In 2008, the STAR was acquired by Small Bone Innovations, Inc. (SBi; Morrisville, PA). The STAR is the only FDA-approved total ankle replacement system intended for uncemented use and is also the only FDA-approved nonconstrained total ankle replacement system. The current SBi STAR implant as described by the current manufacturer has 3 components[13]:

1. Tibial component, available in 5 sizes, with a highly polished flat articular surface and 2 cylindrical fixation bars on the proximal side of the component that anchor the implant to the subchondral bone.
2. Talar component, available in 5 sizes with designation for left and right ankles, with a ridge running anteroposteriorly in the middle of the gliding surface guides of the UHMWPE mobile-bearing sliding core.
3. Mobile-bearing, available in 5 thicknesses of 6 to 10 mm, UHMWPE sliding core, with a flat surface superiorly to articulate with the tibial component and a concave undersurface to articulate the convexity of the talar component and longitudinal ridge.

Regardless, total ankle replacement is a demanding procedure that can ultimately fail for a variety of reasons and require revision. Unfortunately, the scholarly community has yet to form consensus regarding what specifically constitutes a revision of total ankle replacement. As proposed by Henricson and colleagues,[14] current trends are leaning toward using the term *revision* to exclusively indicate removal or exchange of one or more prosthetic components, with the exception of incidental exchange of the UHMWPE insert, thus including ankle arthrodesis and major lower limb amputation. According to this standard, simple UHMWPE exchange and other nonrevision joint-involving secondary surgeries would be considered reoperations. Secondary interventions, such as tibial osteotomies, open reduction internal fixation of fracture, or subtalar joint arthrodesis that do not involve the joint, are considered additional procedures. Ultimately forming consensus and determining a formal definition for *revision* and *failure* of total ankle replacement will aid in understanding survivorship of total ankle replacement, including that of the STAR. Systematic review of the STAR implant has been attempted; however, revision as proposed in this study was neglected, with reoperations and additional procedures not excluded.[8,15,16]

Much debate has existed and published reports vary greatly as to the incidence of failure and revision of the STAR system. According to the inventor, survivorship at 12-year follow-up for the uncemented STAR system is 96%.[17] However, some national registry data, which account for all implantations of total ankle replacement and extractions of failed total ankle replacement within a given country, show that nearly one-third of STAR implants require extraction beyond simple UHMWPE exchange.[18] Thus, to provide clarity and further insight into the revision rate of the uncemented STAR system, involving metallic component exchange, ankle arthrodesis, or major limb amputation, the authors undertook a systematic review.

PATIENTS AND METHODS

Five electronic databases, including the Cochrane Database of Systematic Reviews (http://www.cochrane.org/reviews/; last accessed June 19, 2012); Cochrane Methodology Register (http://cmr.cochrane.org/; last accessed June 19, 2012); Database of Abstracts of Reviews of Effects (http://www.crd.york.ac.uk/crdweb/Home.aspx?DB=DARE; last accessed June 19, 2012); EMBASE (Excerpta Medica database at http://www.embase.com/; last accessed June 19, 2012); and OvidSP Medline (http://ovidsp.tx.ovid.com/; last accessed June 19, 2012) were searched from January 2012 to June 2012, with date restriction from 1990 to present and no restriction regarding language of publication, using an inclusive text word query for "STAR" OR "Scandinavian" AND "total ankle replacement" OR "ankle replacement" OR "ankle arthroplasty" OR "ankle implant" OR "revision surgery" OR "failed surgery," in which the uppercase words represent the Boolean operators used. The references from identified manuscripts were then manually searched for additional potentially pertinent published works, which were then secured for review. Additionally, major podiatric and orthopedic foot and ankle surgery textbooks with chapters on total ankle replacement were obtained to secure any useful material not accessible from the electronic search. Finally, an Internet-based general-interest search engine, specifically Google (http://www.google.com; last accessed June 19, 2012), was used to identify the available sources that could potentially provide useful information, using combinations of the text words listed.

To acquire the highest quality and most relevant studies available, the publications were eligible for inclusion only if they involved patients undergoing primary total ankle replacement with the uncemented STAR system. Accordingly, the search was arbitrarily restricted from January 1990 to present because the STAR system was implanted with cement augmentation before this date. Studies involving both the double-spray porous coating (1990–1999) and single-spray porous coating (2000 to present) were considered for inclusion. The studies additionally required mean follow-up of at least 12 months, a sample size of at least 10 STAR implants, and inclusion of adequate details regarding complications and incidence of revisions (with further stratification of revisions for metallic component exchange, ankle arthrodesis, or major lower limb amputation, and information regarding cause of failure when available). Revision total ankle replacement was defined as 1 of only 3 end points: metallic component exchange, ankle arthrodesis, or amputation proximal to the ankle joint. Reoperations, including isolated UHMWPE mobile-bearing exchanges, and additional procedures were not considered revisions. Reports were not excluded if additional procedures occurred concurrently at the time of index total ankle replacement.

If a reference could not be obtained through purchase, library assistance, or electronic mail contact with the author, it was excluded. If the reference was not written in English, it was translated by the primary author (MAP) from its native language of German or Lithuanian to English using an Internet-based translator, specifically Google Translate (http://translate.google.com/#; last accessed June 19, 2012).

RESULTS

The search for potentially relevant information for inclusion in this systematic review produced a total of 102 reports that underwent rigorous analysis, as detailed in **Fig. 1**, to determine ultimate inclusion. No reports were excluded based on inability to obtain them. Four manuscripts required translation from their native language to English (3 German and 1 Lithuanian), but all of these studies were excluded. However, 1 translated study provided additional information regarding an included study with overlapping patient cohorts.[19] From January to June 2012, the authors reviewed all pertinent references identified, with complete consensus for ultimate inclusion agreed on by the lead author (MAP) and senior author (TSR).

After review of all potentially eligible reports, 20 studies (19.6%) involving true revision of the STAR system (n = 2507) that met inclusion criteria were identified (**Table 1**).[17,18,20–37] In some instances, kin studies were identified that provided additional information to the included works; however, overlap data or insufficient information precluded these studies from ultimate inclusion.[19,38–41] The included studies with available information reported a weighted mean follow-up of 64 months (n = 814; range, 12–156 months). The weighted mean age of patients among the included studies with identifiable data was 62.3 years (n = 1216; range, 22–86 years).

Of the entire study population of 2507 ankles, 269 (10.7%) underwent revision (see **Table 1**). According to the available data, the weighted mean time to revision was 49.7 months (n = 72; range, 1–124 months). Mode of revision was not defined in 139 ankles (51.7% of revisions). One hundred thirty ankles (48.3% of revisions) were identified with a known end point, including 2 amputations (1.5% of known revisions, including 1 below-knee and 1 above-knee amputation), 62 ankle arthrodesis (47.7% of known revisions), and 66 metallic component exchanges (50.8% of known revisions). Of the metallic component exchanges, 33 reported details regarding mode of metallic component revision (50%), whereas the specific revision was indeterminate in 33 metallic component revisions (50%). Of the known metallic component exchanges, 19 were isolated tibial tray exchanges (57.6% of known metallic component exchanges), 4 were isolated talar component exchanges (12.1% of known metallic component exchanges), and 10 were exchanges of both metallic components (30.3% of known metallic component exchanges). Repeat attempts at revision were reported in 5 cases (1.8% of revisions), including 4 metallic component exchange failures that were successfully converted to arthrodesis[19,27,29,32] and 1 ankle arthrodesis that become infected, resulting in concurrent septic arthritis of the ipsilateral total knee replacement that ultimately required conversion to an above-knee amputation.[26] Only

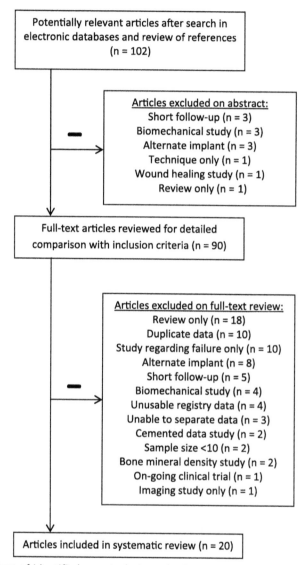

Fig. 1. Flowchart of identified reports during selection process.

index revisions were included, and further revision was not considered as relevant data for the results of this systematic review.

Among the included studies involving registry data from national databases, 798 ankles were identified from 4 reports, and 145 revisions (18.2%) were identified (**Table 2**).[18,23,24,31] Among the registry data, mode of revision was reported in 35 ankles (24.1% of registry revisions), including 0 amputations, 16 ankle arthrodeses (45.7% of known registry revisions), and 19 metallic component exchanges (54.3% of known registry revisions). Of the metallic component exchanges, 11 were isolated tibial tray exchanges (57.9% of known metallic component exchanges), 2 were isolated talar component exchanges (10.5% of known metallic component exchanges),

Table 1
Included studies of systematic review

Investigator	EBM Level	Sample Size STAR (Patients)	Age (y)	F/U (mo) (Range, 12–156)	Revisions (Rate %)	Time to Revision (mo) (Range, 1–124)	Metallic Component Exchange	Ankle Arthrodesis	Amputation	Revisional Procedure Not Reported
Nunley et al,[20] 2012	IV	82 (82)	63.3	61	5 (6.1)	60.7	4	1	0	0
Daniels et al,[21] 2011	IV	113 (99)	NR	46	12 (10.6)	39.5	12	0	0	0
Mann et al,[22] 2011	IV	84 (NR)	61.4	109	8 (9.5)	66.5	3	5	0	0
Rothwell,[a,23] 2011	IV	47 (NR)	NR	>12	7 (14.9)	5.5	0	0	0	7
Henricson et al,[a,18] 2011	IV	322 (NR)	NR	>36	94 (29.2)	52.7	4	16	0	74
Skytta et al,[24] 2010	IV	217 (NR)	NR	>12	29 (13.4)	NR	0	0	0	29
Saltzman et al,[25] 2009	II	596 (NR)	63.1	>24	31 (5.2)	NR	0	1	1 (BKA)	29
ver der Heide et al,[26] 2009	III	37 (NR)	NR	>12	4 (8.1)	NR	0	3	1 (AKA)	0
Hobson et al,[a,27] 2009	IV	123 (111)	64	48	13 (10.6)	NR	9	4	0	0
Wood et al,[28] 2009	III	92 (NR)	65	>36	2 (2.2)	NR	0	2	0	0

Study	EBM									
Wood et al,[29] 2008	IV	200 (NR)	NR	88	23 (11.5)	48	3	20	0	0
Schutte and Louwerens,[30] 2008	IV	49 (47)	57.1	28	4 (8.2)	NR	1	3	0	0
Fevang et al,[31] 2007	IV	212 (NR)	NR	>12	15 (7.1)	NR	15	0	0	0
Kumar and Dhar,[32] 2007	IV	50 (43)	63.3	36	3 (6.0)	NR	2	1	0	0
Kofoed,[17] 2004	IV	25 (25)	58	114	1 (4.0)	96	1	0	0	0
Lodhi et al,[33] 2004	IV	27 (26)	58	>12	1 (3.7)	3	0	1	0	0
Valderrabano et al,[34] 2004	IV	68 (65)	56.1	44	3 (4.4)	NR	3	0	0	0
Schernberg,[35] 1998	IV	131 (NR)	NR	>12	13 (9.9)	NR	9	4	0	0
Huber et al,[36] 1998	IV	12 (12)	NR	>12	1 (8.3)	NR	0	1	0	0
Kofoed and Danborg,[37] 1995	IV	20 (18)	58	30	0 (0.0)	0	0	0	0	0
Total		2507	62.3	64	269 (10.7)	49.7	66	62	2	139

Abbreviations: AKA, above-knee amputation; BKA, below-knee amputation; EBM, evidence based medicine; F/U, follow-up; NR, not reported.
[a] Indicates kin studies were used to provide additional demographic data pertinent to this table.

Table 2
Stratification of data cohorts

Population Subgroup	Sample Size STAR (n)	Number of Revisions	Revision Rate (%)
Entire study cohort[17,18,20–37]	2507	269	10.7
Registry data cohort[18,23,24,31]	798	145	18.2
Cohort excluding inventor/ consultants[18,21,23,24,26–36]	1700	224	13.1
SBi consultant/faculty cohort[20,22,25]	762	44	5.7
Inventor cohort[17,37]	45	1	2.2

Abbreviation: SBi, Small Bone Innovations.

and 6 were exchanges of both metallic components (31.6% of known metallic component exchanges).

Of the included studies involving the inventor as an author, 45 ankles were identified from 2 reports, and 1 revision (2.2%) was identified (see **Table 2**).[17,37] The mode of revision was reported as a metallic component exchange isolated to the tibial tray. No amputations or arthrodeses were reported.

Of the included studies involving known SBi faculty or disclosed consultants, 762 ankles were identified from 3 reports, and 44 revisions (5.7%) were identified (see **Table 2**).[20,22,25] Among the faculty/consultant data, mode of revision was not reported in 29 ankles (65.9% of revisions in this cohort). The mode of revision was reported in 15 ankles (34.1% of faculty/consultant revisions), including 1 below-knee amputation (6.7% of known faculty/consultant revisions), 7 ankle arthrodeses (46.7% of known faculty/consultant revisions), and 7 metallic component exchanges (46.7% of known faculty/consultant revisions). Among the metallic component exchanges, 4 reported details regarding mode of metallic component revision (57.1%), whereas the specific revision was indeterminate in 3 metallic component revisions (42.9%). Among the known metallic component exchanges, 0 were isolated tibial tray exchanges, 1 was an isolated talar component exchange (25% of known metallic component exchanges), and 3 were exchanges of both metallic components (75% of known metallic component exchanges).

Among the included studies except those involving the inventor or SBi faculty or consultants, 1700 ankles were identified from 15 reports, and 224 revisions (13.1%) were identified (see **Table 2**).[18,21,23,24,26–36] Among the worldwide data excluding the inventor and SBi consultants/faculty, mode of revision was not reported in 110 ankles (49.1% of this cohort). The mode of revision was reported in 114 ankles (50.9% of revisions in this cohort), including 1 above-knee amputation (0.9% of known revisions in this cohort), 55 ankle arthrodeses (49.1% of known revisions in this cohort), and 58 metallic component revisions (50.9% of known revisions in this cohort). Among the metallic component exchanges, 28 reported details regarding mode of metallic component revision (48.3%), whereas the specific revision was indeterminate in 30 metallic component revisions (51.7%). Among the known metallic component exchanges, 18 were isolated tibial tray exchanges (64.3% of known metallic component exchanges), 3 were isolated talar component exchanges (10.7% of known metallic component exchanges), and 8 were exchanges of both metallic components (25.0% of known metallic component exchanges).

The specific cause of failure was identified in 183 revisions (68%), whereas the mode of failure was indeterminate in 86 revisions (32%) (**Table 3**). The most common

Table 3
Identified etiology of STAR failure resulting in revision

Cause	Sample Size STAR (n)	Incidence Resulting in Failure (%)
Aseptic loosening	89	48.6
Infection	22	12.0
Technical error	16	8.7
Pain/stiffness	15	8.2
Instability	14	7.7
Fracture	10	5.5
Malalignment	6	3.3
Edge loading	5	2.7
Subsidence	4	2.2
Osteolysis	2	1.1
Total	183	100

cause of failure among included studies was aseptic loosening, which was the reported reason for revision in 89 ankles (48.6% of revisions with known mode of failure). Additional causes included infection (12%), technical error (8.7%), pain/stiffness (8.2%), instability (7.7%), fracture (5.5%), malalignment (3.3%), edge loading (2.7%), subsidence (2.2%), and osteolysis (1.1%).

The methodological quality of the included studies was generally poor. For the 20 studies included, 2 were level 2,[25,28] 1 was level 3,[26] and 17 were level 4 evidence-based medicine studies.[17,18,20–24,27,29–37] Furthermore, of the 20 included studies, 17 (85%) were published in peer-reviewed journals.[17,18,20–22,24–34,37] Four studies (20%) involved data that were obtained from national arthroplasty registries.[18,23,24,31]

DISCUSSION

The purpose of this systematic review was to procure all available quality evidence regarding the incidence of revision after primary implantation of the STAR system. A total of 20 studies involving 2507 ankles with a weighted mean follow-up of 64 months met inclusion criteria. The overall rate of revision was 10.7%. Pooled cohort data of available information revealed that 50.8% of revisions resulted in metallic component exchange, 47.7% resulted in ankle arthrodesis, and 1.5% resulted in major limb amputation.

The results of this systematic review show that the 96% survivorship previously reported by the inventor is not accurate for foot and ankle surgeons as an entity.[17] This high level of survivorship may be attainable for the inventor, who likely has an intimate knowledge of the implant system and its subtleties; however, as shown by this systematic review, this level of success cannot be predictably reproduced among other appropriately trained foot and ankle surgeons. This lack of reproducibility of outcomes was previously shown by Roukis[42] with regard to the Agility Total Ankle Replacement system (DePuy Orthopedics, Inc. Warsaw, IN). In his study, the overall incidence of revision was 9.7% (224/2312); however, excluding the inventor increased the incidence 2-fold, from 6.6% to 12.2%.[42]

Some component of a "learning curve" does seem to be present, as suggested by the inventor, with the implantation of the STAR ankle as a result of complex insertion techniques and intraoperative interpretation of acceptable implant placement.[9,10,17] Wood,[28,29] an experienced STAR surgeon, and colleagues reported an 11.5% revision rate in an initial consecutive series of 200 implanted STAR prostheses, and a 2.2% revision rate in a subsequent series of 92 STAR prostheses. Furthermore, Haskell and Mann[43] noted a 3.1-times greater incidence of perioperative complications in the initial 10 STAR operations compared with the subsequent 10 STAR operations performed by 10 surgeons newly trained in the STAR procedure. However, included studies of this review regarding initial experience reported a pooled 7 revisions in 99 ankles (7.1%) at a weighted mean follow-up of 32 months.[30,32]

The included studies offered a vast range of proposed incidence of revision. Kofoed and Danborg[37] reported a 0% incidence of implant failure requiring revision in one study, whereas Henricson and colleagues[18] noted a 29.2% incidence of failure requiring revision from a national registry data set. However, when removing the cohort data involving the inventor and disclosed consultants of the manufacturer of the implant, the incidence of revision reported increased from 10.7% to 13.1%, whereas the isolated data cohort obtained from registry data reported an 18.2% revision rate.

Registry data help limit the opportunity for patients to be lost to follow-up. When a large subset of patients is lost to follow-up, the incidence of failure may artificially decrease, because patients who are lost to follow-up generally have worse outcomes than patients who continue to be assessed.[44] Registry data secure documentation of further intervention of the total ankle replacement as it occurs and protect against loss to follow-up if a patient seeks care from an alternate surgeon provided the revision is performed in the same country.[45] Several countries throughout Europe and the rest of the world have national joint arthroplasty registries; however, only a limited number of countries currently collect relevant data regarding total ankle replacement. For this systematic review, national registry data from Sweden, Norway, Finland, and New Zealand met inclusion criteria.

The most frequently identified cause of failure was aseptic loosening. Some inconsistencies of terminology were apparent among the included studies. Terms such as *aseptic loosening*, *osteolysis*, and *subsidence* seemed to be used somewhat interchangeably among included studies, which provided difficulty in determining the actual rate of failure for each cause. Further confusion with terminology was noted with the terms *technical error* and *malalignment*.

When the failed STAR implant was amenable to metallic component exchange, the failure occurred at the tibia 57.6% (19 of 33) of the time; whereas failure occurred at the talus only 12.1% (4 of 33) of the time, with the remaining 10 failures occurring at both osseous sites. Frequently, however, failure was not amenable to metallic component exchange, but rather attempted arthrodesis was required. Most studies lacked sufficient detail regarding whether failure occurred at the tibia or talus when arthrodesis was required. Carlsson,[19] however, reported on 20 STAR implants that required revision, with 16 requiring arthrodesis. Of the arthrodeses, 7 (43.8%) were the result of isolated failure of the talus secondary to aseptic loosening. In this cohort, only one failure that occurred at the talus was amenable to metallic component exchange (1 of 8; 12.5%). The STAR frequently may not be amenable to metallic component revision after failure of the talar component, as shown by Carlsson[19]; instead, attempted arthrodesis may be required as a function of product design. The surgical technique, as described by the inventor, requires substantial sculpting to contour the talus to accept the talar component and to aid in realignment and neutralization of the entire hindfoot. Minimum resections of 4 mm from the talar dome and 2 to 3 mm from each the medial and lateral aspects are required, in addition to templated resection of the anterior and posterior portions based on the selected talar component size.[9,10] The benefit of this technique is to correct planar deformity within the mortise of the ankle joint, thus preventing the need for extra-articular realignment. However, when revision is required, much of the talus has already been resected during the primary procedure with removal of nearly all of the dense subchondral bone, which, in addition to possible vascular compromise, may limit structural support, potentially resulting in talar subsidence. The incidence of subsidence and loosening of the talar component may be underreported as a result of limited critical analysis of postoperative radiographs and the design of the talar component, because bony ingrowth is difficult to interpret on plain film radiographs secondary to circumferential metallic artifact.[7,29] The surgical technique and talar component design for primary implantation of the STAR offer limited options when failure of the talus occurs and revision is required. For example, revision options outside of arthrodesis are limited to an UHMWPE exchange to a thicker mobile bearing, exchange of the talar component with or without subtalar joint arthrodesis, or complete extraction with conversion to an alternate total ankle replacement system. Specialized revision components or customizable implants do not appear to be available with the STAR system.

Rigorous analysis of serial postoperative radiographs has been proposed when loosening or impending failure is suspected. Five millimeters or more of subsidence of the talar component on the lateral view is considered indicative for loosening. Meanwhile, angular change of either component greater than 5° in any plane has been suggested as evidence for migration and/or subsidence. Although beyond the scope of this review, Bestic and colleagues[7] proposed several angular measurements to aid in monitoring and evaluating postoperative progression of total ankle replacement (**Table 4**).

Weaknesses of this systematic review can be identified. First, it only evaluated revision of primary implantation of STAR defined by failure resulting in metallic component exchange, ankle arthrodesis, or major amputation of a lower limb. Reoperations and

Table 4
Radiographic measurements for postoperative evaluation of total ankle replacement

Title of Measurement	Definition
α	On the anterior-posterior view of the ankle, the α angle is formed by the intersection of the lines drawn to the flat plate of the tibial component and the long axis of the tibial shaft (normal = 90°).
β	On the lateral view of the ankle, the β angle is formed by the intersection of the lines drawn parallel to the flat plate of the tibial component and the long axis of the tibial shaft (normal = 90°).
γ	The γ angle is formed by the intersection of a line drawn through the long axis of the talar component with a line drawn from the posterior talar component through the middle of the talar neck (range = 1.1°–33.4°, average = 18.8°).
a	The "a" measurement is the perpendicular distance between the tip of the lateral malleolus and a line drawn through the base of the tibial component on the anterior-posterior view.
b	The "b" measurement is the perpendicular distance from the anterior aspect of the talar component to a line intersecting the calcaneal tubercle and dorsal aspect of the talo-navicular joint on the lateral view.
c	The "c" measurement is the perpendicular distance from the posterior aspect of the talar component to a line intersecting the calcaneal tubercle and dorsal aspect of the talo-navicular joint.

From Bestic JM, Bancroft LW, Peterson JJ, et al. Postoperative imaging of the total ankle arthroplasty. Radiol Clin N Am 2008;46:1003–15; with permission.

additional procedures were not considered as revisions; however, this is not to say that these do not result in increased morbidity and that they should be overlooked, but rather this was done to provide an accurate assessment of the rate of revision for primary implantation of the STAR implant. Second, procurement of pertinent reports was obtained via electronic database search, and therefore further studies may exist that were overlooked, inadvertently excluded, or simply not identified by the methods used. Next, 3 of the 20 included studies were not subjected to the rigors of the peer review process. Furthermore, 4 reports involved data that were obtained from national arthroplasty registry databases; however, 3 of these included reports were obtained from previously published peer reviewed manuscripts. Additionally, the use of a readily available online translation program was used to translate non-English manuscripts, which may have introduced bias; however, this process was performed similarly to that in previously published works, and no translated studies were included as a stand-alone resource but rather as a cohort overlap supplement to an already included study.[42] Finally, of the included 20 reports, not all studies included all demographic data evaluated; accordingly, weighted means were formulated based on all available information, with sample sizes indicated for each.

Currently, 4 ankle prostheses are FDA-approved for implantation in the United States. The STAR implant is the only nonconstrained mobile-bearing implant available, whereas the other 3, Agility LP Total Ankle System (DePuy Orthopedics, Inc. Warsaw, IN), INBONE and INBONE II (Wright Medical Technologies, Inc. Arlington, TN), and Salto-Talaris (Tornier, Inc. Edina, MN), are 2-component fixed-bearing implant systems. Understanding survivorship, potential modes of failure, and options for revision of failed implant replacement are paramount to selecting the appropriate ankle prosthesis for a given patient and ankle condition.

In conclusion, a systematic review of available data regarding primary implantation of the uncemented STAR implant showed the incidence of revision to be 10.7%. When excluding the inventor and disclosed consultants of the current manufacturer, the incidence of revision increased to 13.1%. Finally, data isolated to the national joint arthroplasty registries showed an 18.2% incidence of revision. Because most included level 4 evidence-based medicine studies, further appropriately weighted cohort studies with comparison groups, prospective studies, and continued evaluation using national joint arthroplasty registries are warranted, in addition to direct comparison of the STAR system with other commonly used contemporary total ankle replacement systems.

REFERENCES

1. Vickerstaff JA, Miles AW, Cunningham JL. A brief history of total ankle replacement and a review of the current status. Med Eng Phys 2007;29:1056–64.
2. Coughlin MJ. The Scandinavian total ankle replacement prosthesis. Instr Course Lect 2002;51:135–42.
3. Gittins J, Mann RA. The history of the STAR total ankle arthroplasty. Foot Ankle Clin 2002;7:809–16.
4. Easley ME, Vertullo CJ, Urban WC, et al. Total ankle arthroplasty. J Am Acad Orthop Surg 2002;10:157–67.
5. Guyer AJ, Richardson EG. Current concepts review: total ankle arthroplasty. Foot Ankle Int 2008;29(2):256–64.
6. Easley ME, Adams SB Jr, Hembree C, et al. Current concepts review: results of total ankle arthroplasty. J Bone Joint Surg Am 2011;93-A:1455–68.
7. Bestic JM, Bancroft LW, Peterson JJ, et al. Postoperative imaging of the total ankle arthroplasty. Radiol Clin North Am 2008;46:1003–15.

8. Zhao H, Yang Y, Yu G, et al. A systematic review of outcome and failure rate of uncemented Scandinavian total ankle replacement. Int Orthop 2011;35:1751–8.
9. Kofoed H. Scandinavian total ankle replacement: the surgical technique. Tech Foot Ankle Surg 2005;4(1):55–61.
10. Kofoed H. Concept and use of the Scandinavian total ankle replacement. Foot Ankle Spec 2009;2(2):89–94.
11. Wood PL. Experience with the STAR ankle arthroplasty at Wrightington Hospital, UK. Foot Ankle Clin 2002;7:755–64.
12. U.S. Food and Drug Administration. Approval Order for Scandinavian Total Ankle Replacement System (STAR Ankle). Available at: http://www.accessdata.fda.gov/cdrh_docs/pdf5/p050050a.pdf. Accessed June 6, 2012.
13. Small Bone Innovations. STAR. Available at: http://www.star-ankle.com/. Accessed June 19, 2012.
14. Henricson A, Carlsson A, Rydholm U. What is a revision of total ankle arthroplasty? Foot Ankle Surg 2011;17:99–102.
15. Gougoulias N, Khanna A, Maffulli N. How successful are current ankle replacements? Clin Orthop Relat Res 2010;468(1):199–208.
16. Glazebrook MA, Arsenault K, Dunbar M. Evidence-based classification of complications in total ankle arthroplasty. Foot Ankle Int 2009;30(10):945–9.
17. Kofoed H. Scandinavian total ankle replacement (STAR). Clin Orthop Relat Res 2004;424:73–9.
18. Henricson A, Nilsson JA, Carlsson A. 10-year survival of total ankle arthroplasties. Acta Orthop 2011;82(6):655–9.
19. Carlsson A. Einfach-und doppeltbeschictete STAR-Sprunggelenkprothesen. Orthopade 2006;35:527–32 [in German].
20. Nunley JA, Caputo AM, Easley ME, et al. Intermediate to long-term outcomes of the STAR total ankle replacement: the patient perspective. J Bone Joint Surg Am 2012;94:43–8.
21. Daniels TR, Penner MJ, Mayich DJ, et al. Prospective clinical and radiographic intermediate outcomes of 113 Scandinavian total ankle arthroplasties. J Bone Joint Surg Br 2011;93(Supp IV):584.
22. Mann JA, Mann RA, Horton E. STAR Ankle: long-term results. Foot Ankle Int 2011; 32(5):473–84.
23. Rothwell AG. The New Zealand joint registry twelve-year report. Available at: http://www.cdhb.govt.nz/njr/reports/A2D65CA3.pdf. Accessed June 20, 2012.
24. Skytta ET, Koivu H, Ikävalko M, et al. Total ankle replacement: a population-based study of 515 cases from the Finnish arthroplasty register. Acta Orthop 2010;81(1): 114–8.
25. Saltzman CL, Mann RA, Ahrens JE, et al. Prospective controlled trial of STAR total ankle replacement versus ankle fusion: initial results. Foot Ankle Int 2009;30(7): 579–96.
26. van der Heide HJ, Schutte B, Louwerens JW, et al. Total ankle prostheses in rheumatoid arthropathy. Acta Orthop 2009;80(4):440–4.
27. Hobson SA, Karantana A, Dhar S. Total ankle replacement in patients with significant pre-operative deformity of the hindfoot. J Bone Joint Surg Br 2009;91(4):481–6.
28. Wood PL, Sutton C, Mishra V, et al. A randomized, controlled trial of two mobile-bearing total ankle replacements. J Bone Joint Surg Br 2009;91(1):69–74.
29. Wood PL, Prem H, Sutton C. Total ankle replacement: medium term results in 200 Scandinavian Total Ankle Replacements. J Bone Joint Surg Br 2008;90(5):605–9.
30. Schutte BG, Louwerens JW. Short-term results of our first 49 Scandinavian Total Ankle Replacements (STAR). Foot Ankle Int 2008;29(2):124–7.

31. Fevang BT, Lie SA, Havelin LI, et al. 257 ankle arthroplasties performed in Norway between 1994 and 2005. Acta Orthop 2007;78(5):575–83.
32. Kumar A, Dhar S. Total ankle replacement: early results during learning period. Foot Ankle Surg 2007;13:19–23.
33. Lodhi Y, McKenna C, Herron M, et al. Total ankle replacement. Ir Med J 2004; 97(4):104–5.
34. Valderrabano V, Hintermann B, Dick W. Scandinavian Total Ankle Replacement: a 3.7 year average follow-up of 65 patients. Clin Orthop Relat Res 2004;424: 47–56.
35. Schernberg F. Current results of ankle arthroplasty—European multi-center study of cementless ankle arthroplasty. In: Hakon Kofoed, editor. Current status of ankle arthroplasty. Berlin: Kofoed; 1998. p. 41–6.
36. Huber H, Kellenberger R, Huber M. Scandinavian Total Ankle Replacement (LINK S.T.A.R.): technical problems and solutions. In: Hakon Kofoed, editor. Current status of ankle arthroplasty. Berlin: Kofoed; 1998. p. 106–10.
37. Kofoed H, Danborg L. Biological fixation of ankle arthroplasty. Foot 1995;5:27–31.
38. Hosman AH, Mason RB, Hobbs T, et al. A New Zealand national joint registry review of 202 total ankle replacements followed for up to 6 years. Acta Orthop 2007;78(5):584–91.
39. Karantana A, Hobson S, Dhar S. The Scandinavian total ankle replacement. Clin Orthop Relat Res 2009;468:951–7.
40. Anderson T, Montgomery F, Carlsson A. Uncemented STAR total ankle prostheses: surgical technique. J Bone Joint Surg Am 2004;86(Suppl I):103–11.
41. Henricson A, Agren PH. Secondary surgery after total ankle replacement: the influence of preoperative hindfoot alignment. Foot Ankle Surg 2007;13:41–4.
42. Roukis TS. Incidence of revision after primary implantation of the Agility total ankle replacement system: a systematic review. J Foot Ankle Surg 2012;51: 198–204.
43. Haskell A, Mann RA. Perioperative complication rate of total ankle replacement is reduced by surgeon experience. Foot Ankle Int 2004;25(5):283–9.
44. Murray DW, Britton AR, Bulstrode CJ. Loss to follow-up matters. J Bone Joint Surg Br 1997;79(2):254–7.
45. Hyer CF, Portera WB, Haglund EM. Lower extremity implant registries: has the time come in the United States? Foot Ankle Spec 2010;3(3):148–52.

Current Concepts and Techniques in Foot and Ankle Surgery

Concomitant Osteomyelitis and Avascular Necrosis of the Talus Treated with Talectomy and Tibiocalcaneal Arthrodesis

John J. Stapleton, DPM[a,b], Thomas Zgonis, DPM[c],*

KEYWORDS

- Avascular necrosis • Osteomyelitis • Charcot foot • Neuropathy • Talus
- External fixation

KEY POINTS

- The incidence of avascular necrosis from a complex talus fracture is high.
- External fixation use for talectomy and tibiocalcaneal arthrodesis can provide successful outcomes in the presence of soft tissue and/or defects.
- Single or staged talectomy with a tibiocalcaneal arthrodesis depends on but is not limited to the patient's history, medical optimization, clinical presentation, laboratory findings, and medical imaging.
- A multidisciplinary team approach is crucial for the patient's overall successful outcome.

INTRODUCTION

The use of external fixation to perform lower extremity salvage arthrodesis in the presence of osseous and/or soft-tissue infection is a valuable tool that allows adequate osseous realignment and stability while avoiding the insertion of retained implants that can act as a nidus for latent or recurrent infection. Permanent cemented antibiotic-impregnated hindfoot intramedullary nails have also been used to achieve arthrodesis of the hindfoot/ankle in the presence of talar osteomyelitis and avascular necrosis (AVN).[1–4]

In this article, the following clinical case scenarios demonstrate the use of circular external fixation to treat complex talar fractures complicated with AVN, structural

[a] Foot and Ankle Surgery, VSAS Orthopaedics, Lehigh Valley Hospital, 1250 South Cedar Crest Boulevard, Suite #110, Allentown, PA 18103, USA; [b] Department of Surgery, Penn State College of Medicine, 500 University Drive, Hershey, PA 17033, USA; [c] Division of Podiatric Medicine and Surgery, Department of Orthopaedic Surgery, University of Texas Health Science Center at San Antonio, 7703 Floyd Curl Drive, MSC 7776, San Antonio, TX 78229, USA
* Corresponding author.
E-mail address: zgonis@uthscsa.edu

Clin Podiatr Med Surg 30 (2013) 251–256
http://dx.doi.org/10.1016/j.cpm.2013.01.001
0891-8422/13/$ – see front matter © 2013 Elsevier Inc. All rights reserved.

collapse, and infection with a single-stage talectomy and tibiocalcaneal arthrodesis and how staged procedures are more commonly used in the management of diabetic Charcot neuroarthropathy. The dilemma arises as to whether a single or staged procedure is required when performing a septic tibiocalcaneal arthrodesis. The first clinical case scenario demonstrates a single-stage talectomy and tibiocalcaneal arthrodesis for the management of posttraumatic talar AVN and concomitant osteomyelitis. However, diabetic patients with Charcot neuroarthropathy and concomitant talar osteomyelitis are typically treated with a staged talectomy and tibiocalcaneal arthrodesis. The clinical presentation of infected ulcerations, active drainage, and the presence of purulence when managing the diabetic patient with Charcot neuroarthropathy is surgically approached with a multiple-staged reconstruction to achieve a successful tibiocalcaneal arthrodesis.

CLINICAL CASE SCENARIOS

In the first clinical case scenario, the patient presented with a history of severe pain in the right ankle after developing AVN of the talus that led to a collapse and posttraumatic deformity. The patient's past medical history was significant for pulmonary embolism 20 years prior, a history of alcohol abuse, and a 30-pack-year history of smoking tobacco. The patient reported a sustained complex talus neck and body fracture with a concomitant ankle fracture to the ipsilateral extremity after a fall from a roof. An open reduction and internal fixation of the talus, lateral malleolus, and syndesmosis was performed at the time of injury. In the initial postoperative period, the patient reported difficulty with healing of the medial surgical incision secondary to wound dehiscence. Treatment at that time consisted of local wound care and oral antibiotics until the surgical wound was healed. Six months from the initial surgery the patient had internal fixation hardware removal from the lateral malleolus and syndesmosis injury. The patient was permitted to increased weight-bearing status and eventually developed posttraumatic collapse of the avascular talus and nonunion of the ankle that led to severe valgus deformity.

The neurovascular status of the affected lower extremity was intact. The surgical incisions were also healed in the presence of moderate edema and surrounding post-inflammatory hyperpigmentation and scar contractures. There was no open wound or evidence of a draining sinus. A fixed hindfoot and ankle valgus deformity was evident, and the patient was unable to ambulate for activities of daily living. A chronic infectious process was suspected but not confirmed by laboratory or nuclear imaging studies. The results of all laboratory tests were within normal limits, and a white blood cell labeled bone scan with a 24-hour delay could not confirm deep infection or osteomyelitis.

Surgical treatment options discussed with the patient included a single and/or staged talectomy with a tibiocalcaneal arthrodesis versus a lower extremity amputation. Based on the preoperative laboratory and medical imaging testing, a single-stage talectomy and tibiocalcaneal arthrodesis with a circular external fixator was performed. Intraoperatively, 2 bone cultures from the talus were obtained along with 1 bone culture from the lateral malleolus. All bone that was resected was also sent for histopathologic analysis. The 2 bone cultures from the talus identified methicillin-sensitive *Staphylococcus aureus*, whereas the histopathologic analysis from the talus was positive for osteomyelitis. Infectious disease consultation was initiated, and medical management consisted of a 10-week course of oral minocycline, 100 mg, twice daily. Postoperatively, the patient was kept non–weight bearing with the circular external fixator for approximately 6 weeks. At that time, all wounds were healed and the provisional Steinmann pins were removed, whereas the external fixator was modified by attaching a postoperative shoe that allowed the patient to begin partial weight bearing as tolerated. The external fixator was removed at 12 weeks postoperation. The patient first had a walking cast for an additional 4 weeks and then progressed to wearing a shoe with a lift to accommodate for the 3.5-cm limb length discrepancy. At 1-year follow-up, the patient demonstrated successful arthrodesis with no evidence of recurrent infection (**Fig. 1**).

Similarly, in cases with a severe fracture dislocation of the diabetic Charcot neuroarthropathy hindfoot and ankle with or without concomitant osteomyelitis, a 1-stage versus staged talectomy and tibiocalcaneal arthrodesis is performed for osseous and soft-tissue reconstruction. In the presence of large soft-tissue defects with or without osteomyelitis, circular external fixation becomes ideal for lower extremity limb salvage. As described earlier, necessary preoperative and intraoperative laboratory and medical imaging becomes crucial to the surgeon's decision between salvage arthrodesis and lower extremity amputation.

In the diabetic patient with Charcot neuroarthropathy, confirmed osteomyelitis of the talus is most commonly treated with serial surgical debridements, cemented antibiotic impregnated spacers, beads, and staged talectomy with tibiocalcaneal arthrodesis. Internal fixation is usually avoided but may be used when clean surgical osseous and soft-tissue margins are obtained after serial surgical debridements and the patient has completed a prolonged course of antibiotic therapy as directed and monitored by an infectious disease specialist with an interest in diabetic lower extremity pathology and reconstruction. A 1-stage talectomy and tibiocalcaneal arthrodesis is also indicated in the diabetic patient with Charcot neuroarthropathy when there is no history of open wounds or infections in the lower extremity or when the patient presents with a soft-tissue defect but without any evidence of a talar osteomyelitis. Adjunctive therapies including but not limited to negative pressure wound therapy, bone grafting, biologic dressings, and hyperbaric oxygen therapy may also be used in the diabetic patient with Charcot neuroarthropathy (**Fig. 2**).

In both clinical case scenarios, it is important to emphasize the role of the multidisciplinary team approach for the patient's overall successful outcome. Obtaining a detailed and extensive past medical history, laboratory testing, medical imaging, and vascular evaluation and testing in addition to the patient's medical optimization are all important factors in the final diagnosis and surgical treatment of these complex injuries. Intraoperative soft-tissue and osseous cultures, bone biopsy, and histopathologic analysis may later reveal an infectious process as presented with the first clinical case scenario described earlier. A high index of suspicion is paramount with a history of talar AVN related to complicated traumatic wounds or in cases of Charcot neuroarthropathy of the hindfoot/ankle.

DISCUSSION

In the first clinical case scenario, circular external fixation was chosen for the 1-stage talectomy with tibiocalcaneal arthrodesis for several reasons. First, despite a negative preoperative infectious workup with necessary testing, chronic deep infection was still clinically suspected according to the patient's history and clinical presentation. Second, lower extremity deformity correction and postoperative adjustments could have been made with an external fixation device to achieve the desired alignment and successful arthrodesis, and last, circular external fixation could have allowed for earlier weight-bearing status and closer monitoring of the surgical incisions.

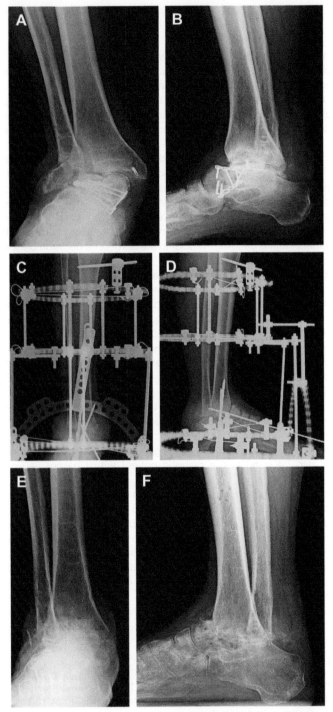

Fig. 1. Preoperative anteroposterior and lateral ankle radiographs (*A, B*) showing the avascular necrosis of the talus with collapse and nonunion of the lateral malleolus with significant valgus deformity and loss of talar height after an open reduction and internal fixation. Postoperative anteroposterior and lateral ankle radiographs (*C, D*) at 2 weeks showing the tibiocalcaneal arthrodesis alignment in 1-stage talectomy with circular external fixation. Postoperative anteroposterior and lateral ankle radiographs (*E, F*) at 1-year follow-up demonstrating successful alignment and union of the tibiocalcaneal arthrodesis.

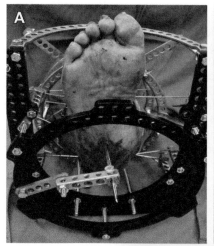

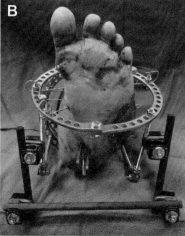

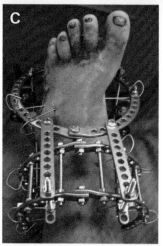

Fig. 2. Clinical case examples using circular external fixation for staged talectomy with tibio-calcaneal arthrodesis procedures in the diabetic patient with Charcot neuroarthropathy. Note the 2 different circular external fixation devices with incorporated Steinmann pin fixation to the external fixation plate (*A*) and locked ankle hinged devices with a forefoot circular ring (*B, C*).

The surgical decision in the diabetic patient with Charcot neuroarthropathy is multifactorial and depends on the patient's overall medical condition, associated comorbidities, presence of soft-tissue infection or osteomyelitis, severity of fracture, dislocation and AVN of the talus, ambulatory status, peripheral vascular disease, body mass index, patient's compliance with medical and surgical treatments, and social support.

Surgical experience for these complex conditions becomes paramount, as latent infections, nonunions, and wound healing complications can lead to lower extremity amputation. The use of circular external fixation among these difficult-to-treat clinical case scenarios may allow for a single or staged reconstruction with a talectomy and tibiocalcaneal arthrodesis. Further studies comparing single versus staged talectomy and tibiocalcaneal arthrodesis among these clinical scenarios is required.

REFERENCES

1. Facaros Z, Ramanujam CL, Stapleton JJ. Combined circular external fixation and open reduction internal fixation with pro-syndesmotic screws for repair of a diabetic ankle fracture. Diabet Foot Ankle 2010;1:5554.
2. Stapleton JJ, Zgonis T. Surgical reconstruction of the diabetic Charcot foot: internal, external or combined fixation? Clin Podiatr Med Surg 2012;29:425–33.
3. Ramanujam CL, Zgonis T. Antibiotic-loaded cement beads for Charcot ankle osteomyelitis. Foot Ankle Spec 2010;3:274–7.
4. Woods JB, Lowery NJ, Burns PR. Permanent antibiotic impregnated intramedullary nail in diabetic limb salvage: a case report and literature review. Diabet Foot Ankle 2012;3:11908.

Diabetic Lisfranc Fracture-Dislocations and Charcot Neuroarthropathy

Bradley A. Levitt, DPM[a], John J. Stapleton, DPM[b,c],
Thomas Zgonis, DPM[a,*]

KEYWORDS

- Lisfranc joint • Fracture • Charcot neuroarthropathy • External fixation
- Diabetes mellitus

KEY POINTS

- Considerations affecting the choice of procedure include the patient's overall medical status, fracture pattern, open versus closed injuries, osseous deformity, compartment syndrome, neurovascular status, and associated soft tissue compromise.
- Open reduction and internal fixation is usually performed when closed reduction with percutaneous fixation is unable to reduce the associated deformity.
- Primary arthrodesis may be considered in severe Lisfranc fracture-dislocations and in diabetic patients with dense peripheral neuropathy.
- External fixation provides a method of fracture reduction with limited compromise to the soft tissue envelope and can be used as a temporary or definitive method of fixation in the diabetic neuropathic population with Lisfranc fracture-dislocation.

INTRODUCTION

Appropriate management of Lisfranc injuries among the general population has been well documented in the literature but little information exists on treatment modification for the diabetic population. Missed and/or conservative treatment options have been found to result in poor long-term outcomes, mostly leading to midfoot instability, chronic pain, and posttraumatic arthrosis.[1] Early studies in the surgical treatment of Lisfranc fracture-dislocations have reported successful outcomes with anatomic alignment and open reduction techniques.[2] Some of the most common surgical options include closed reduction with percutaneous fixation, open reduction with

[a] Division of Podiatric Medicine and Surgery, Department of Orthopaedic Surgery, University of Texas Health Science Center at San Antonio, 7703 Floyd Curl Drive MSC 7776, San Antonio, TX 78229, USA; [b] Foot and Ankle Surgery, VSAS Orthopaedics, Lehigh Valley Hospital, 1250 South Cedar Crest Boulevard, Suite # 110, Allentown, PA 18103, USA; [c] Department of Surgery, Penn State College of Medicine, 500 University Drive, Hershey, PA 17033, USA
* Corresponding author.
E-mail address: zgonis@uthscsa.edu

Clin Podiatr Med Surg 30 (2013) 257–263
http://dx.doi.org/10.1016/j.cpm.2013.01.002
0891-8422/13/$ – see front matter © 2013 Elsevier Inc. All rights reserved.

internal fixation, primary arthrodesis, and external fixation. Considerations affecting the choice of procedure include the patient's overall medical status, fracture type/ pattern, open versus closed injuries, osseous deformity, compartment syndrome, neurovascular status, and associated soft tissue injuries. The objective in the diabetic patient with confounding peripheral neuropathy is to regain and maintain stability in the midfoot. Delay in diagnosis and treatment can predispose the diabetic neuropathic patient to ulcerate, develop an infection, or Charcot neuroarthropathy with potential amputation in some cases.[3]

INITIAL EVALUATION AND DIAGNOSIS

A thorough history and physical examination can reveal common findings raising the index of suspicion for Lisfranc fracture-dislocation. Specific mechanisms of injury have been described that typically correlate with these types of injuries, including direct trauma from an axial load to the involved foot, a fall from a height, or a crush injury leading to multiple comminuted fractures. Other mechanisms include indirect trauma associated with eversion/pronation or hyperplantarflexed digits with a non–weight-bearing hindfoot.[4,5] Regardless of the mechanism of injury, accurate anatomic reduction and stability across the tarsometatarsal joints have been shown to be reliable factors associated with a successful outcome for the patient.[6]

Physical examination findings typically consist of pain over the region of dislocation/ fracture, pain with passive forefoot pronation/supination, plantar medial arch edema, and ecchymosis.[7,8] In the diabetic population, the history and physical examination may be increasingly inconclusive, especially when accompanied by dense peripheral neuropathy. In most cases, the diabetic patient may present with no recollection of sustaining any injury. The history and physical examination should also identify any other risk factors that may alter the procedure selection such as the detection of peripheral arterial disease, peripheral neuropathy, and associated medical comorbidities. In addition, surgical emergencies such as compartment syndrome, acute vascular compromise, open fractures, and/or severe dislocations, may still need to be addressed.

Plain radiographic evaluation consists of anteroposterior, oblique, and lateral foot and/or ankle/lower extremity films if indicated. The presence of metatarsal base(s) and/or associated tarsal fractures raises the concern for a Lisfranc injury. The plain radiographic diagnosis consists of increased diastasis (usually >2 mm) between the first and second metatarsals and/or tarsometatarsal joint incongruity, but in some cases, plain radiographs alone are not enough to make a diagnosis.[9] Because most plain radiographs in the acute setting are performed in a non–weight-bearing situation, the diastasis, ligamentous injuries, and/or tarsometatarsal incongruity may not be evident; the close proximity of the bones can cause significant overlapping, which can make subtle fractures difficult to identify.

Other medical imaging modalities to consider with this type of injury include stress radiographs, magnetic resonance imaging (MRI), and computed tomography (CT). Stress radiographs can detect joint subluxation by applying abduction/pronation and adduction/supination across the tarsometatarsal joints. MRI allows for visualization of the ligamentous complex and the presence of any disruption or attenuation can be determined.[10] In the diabetic population, MRI may also detect early neuropathic changes accompanying the initial Lisfranc fracture-dislocation. Both MRI and stress foot radiographs are useful in cases where obvious fracture and/or dislocation are not present. CT can accurately delineate the fracture pattern to assist in surgical reduction and procedure selection.

TREATMENT

Conservative treatment is usually not used in the management of traumatic Lisfranc fracture-dislocations and may lead to significant osseous deformity, chronic pain, and posttraumatic arthrosis. Conservative treatments rely on reconstitution of the ligamentous structures with prolonged immobilization as the means of maintaining tarsometatarsal joint congruity. Serial plain radiographs are required for evaluation of any instability and/or development of incongruity at the level of the midfoot. This treatment approach may be used in certain patients with minor injuries or minimal diastasis and instability and/or in patients who are not surgical candidates.

With open reduction and internal or percutaneous fixation, close attention must be paid to the soft tissue envelope due to the necessity of multiple surgical incisions. After open reduction is achieved, internal fixation is performed using screw(s), wire(s), and/or plate(s) fixation (**Fig. 1**). The eventual removal of the fixation relies on reestablishing healing of the surrounding soft tissues and ligamentous attachments to maintain the structural integrity of the foot. This procedural approach requires careful consideration of wound-healing potential. Diabetic patients with any degree of peripheral vascular disease who require multiple incisions that entail narrow skin bridges may be predisposed to eventual skin necrosis. In the diabetic population, surgical management of Lisfranc fracture-dislocation is dependent on but not limited by the fracture pattern, past medical history, associated comorbidities, peripheral vascular disease, presence of peripheral neuropathy, and ambulatory status (**Figs. 2** and **3**).

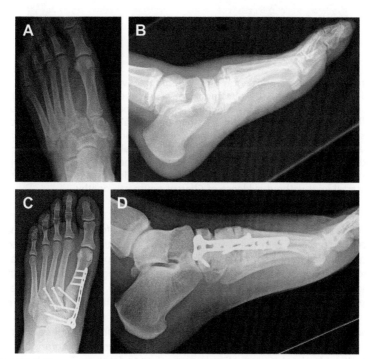

Fig. 1. Preoperative anteroposterior (A) and lateral (B) radiographic views showing a Lisfranc fracture-dislocation variant extending into the naviculocuneiform joints as a result of a motorcycle accident. Postoperative anteroposterior (C) and lateral (D) radiographic views showing anatomic reduction and use of a medial column bridge plate.

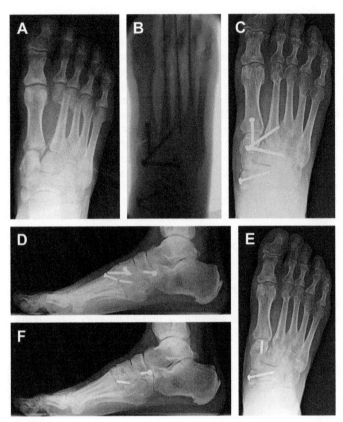

Fig. 2. Preoperative anteroposterior (*A*) radiographic view demonstrating a Lisfranc fracture-dislocation variant with concomitant navicular and multiple metatarsal neck fractures as a result of a motor vehicle accident. The patient's past medical history included diabetes mellitus, peripheral neuropathy, and mild peripheral arterial disease. Intraoperative anteroposterior (*B*), postoperative anteroposterior (*C*), and lateral (*D*) radiographic views demonstrating successful anatomic reduction with minimally open and percutaneous fixation. Hardware removal was performed after 6 months and postoperative anteroposterior (*E*) and lateral (*F*) radiographs at 1 year demonstrated mild posttraumatic arthrosis at the tarsometatarsal joint without evidence of Charcot neuroarthropathy.

The role of primary arthrodesis for pure ligamentous Lisfranc joint injuries has been studied and compared with outcomes after open reduction and internal fixation.[11] Primary arthrodesis may also be useful in the diabetic population with dense peripheral neuropathy to provide osseous union to maintain long-term stability in the midfoot. Traditionally, this procedure had been performed as a salvage method or when severe joint comminution or entire joint dislocation has occurred as a result of injury.

External fixation provides a method of fracture reduction with limited compromise to the soft tissue envelope. This modality can be used as a temporary or definitive fixation method for fracture reduction in case of open fracture. The external fixation device can be inserted outside the zone of injury so that contaminated and/or infected areas can be treated with antibiotic beads/spacers and large wounds can be treated with negative-pressure wound therapy with subsequent closure.[12,13] In addition, in

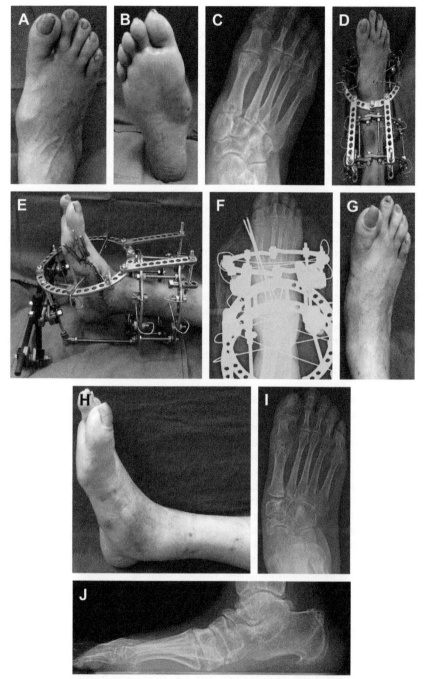

Fig. 3. Preoperative clinical (*A, B*) and anteroposterior (*C*) radiographic views showing a chronic diabetic Charcot neuroarthropathy at the Lisfranc joint with a history of Lisfranc joint dislocation many years previously. The patient underwent a staged reconstruction with an initial surgical debridement, wide ulcer excision and subsequent medial column arthrodesis, and rearfoot/ankle stabilization with the use of a circular external fixator (*D–F*). The external fixation system was removed at approximately 7 weeks. Final postoperative clinical (*G, H*) and radiographic (*I, J*) views at approximately 1-year follow-up.

diabetic patients with less than optimal vasculature supply to the lower extremity, external fixation can provide reduction and long-term stability requiring only percutaneous incisions. External fixation can also be used in combination with internal fixation for enhanced stability in primary arthrodesis or in the initial reduction of deformity and further stabilization of proximal rearfoot/ankle joints when necessary.[14]

Whether an operative or nonoperative treatment is used, the diabetic neuropathic patient recovering from a Lisfranc fracture-dislocation requires close outpatient follow-up and monitoring. Serial plain radiographic evaluation is necessary to check for evidence of midfoot instability requiring shoe modifications and/or bracing versus subsequent operative procedures. Further structural changes from diabetic posttraumatic deformity, nonunion, and collapse may contribute to the development of ulceration, infection, and Charcot neuroarthropathy.[15]

Gross instability at the diabetic Lisfranc joint compounded by peripheral neuropathy, although rarely reported in the literature, may precipitate the development of Charcot neuroarthropathy.[3] The advent of an unstable and/or surgically induced Charcot neuroarthropathy of the Lisfranc joint will most likely require extensive reconstruction by revision surgery, which may include joint arthrodesis along with soft tissue manipulation (tendo-Achilles lengthening vs gastrocnemius recession) to reestablish a stable plantigrade foot. To date no specific guidelines have been reported to specifically address surgical fixation and approach to Lisfranc injuries in diabetic patients. Limited literature is available on the management and complications of diabetic ankle fractures. Although variation exists in treatment methods and protocols, the general consensus is that increased methods of fixation, avoidance of early fixation removal, and longer periods of immobilization are necessary for the diabetic population.[16–18]

Complications arising from Lisfranc fracture-dislocations in the diabetic population exist on multiple levels.[15] In addition to the presence of several medical comorbidities associated with the diabetic patient, hyperglycemia serves as an immunosuppressant, predisposing the patient to the development of subsequent infections.[19] Diabetic patients with peripheral arterial disease may also run the risk of soft tissue necrosis and complications caused by lack of blood flow. These complications may require a decision on the need for revascularization versus amputation in severe cases of Lisfranc injuries. Careful patient selection and surgical experience with these types of injuries can help guide the treatment to provide a successful outcome for the patient.

This review article has emphasized the unique presentation of Lisfranc fracture-dislocations in the diabetic population. Further studies are necessary to evaluate treatment protocols and fixation methods for diabetic patients with dense peripheral neuropathy and/or associated peripheral vascular disease.

REFERENCES

1. Aronow MS. Treatment of the missed Lisfranc injury. Foot Ankle Clin 2006;11: 127–42.
2. Myerson MS, Fisher RT, Burgess AR, et al. Fracture dislocations of the tarsometatarsal joints: end results correlated with pathology and treatment. Foot Ankle 1986;6:225–42.
3. Yeoh J, Muir KR, Dissanayake AM, et al. Lisfranc fracture-dislocation precipitating acute Charcot arthropathy in a neuropathic diabetic foot: a case report. Cases J 2008;1:290.
4. Kalia V, Fishman EK, Carrino JA, et al. Epidemiology, imaging, and treatment of Lisfranc fracture-dislocations revisited. Skeletal Radiol 2012;41:129–36.

5. van der Werf GJ, Tonino AJ. Tarsometatarsal fracture-dislocation. Acta Orthop Scand 1984;55:647–51.

6. Hardcastle PH, Reschauer R, Kutscha-Lissberg E, et al. Injuries to the tarsome-tatarsal joint. Incidence, classification and treatment. J Bone Joint Surg Br 1982; 64:349–56.

7. Rhim B, Hunt JC. Lisfranc injury and Jones fractures in sports. Clin Podiatr Med Surg 2011;28:69–86.

8. Ross G, Cronin R, Hauzenblas J, et al. Plantar ecchymosis sign: a clinical aid to diagnosis of occult Lisfranc tarsometatarsal injuries. J Orthop Trauma 1996;10: 119–22.

9. Sherief TI, Mucci B, Greiss M. Lisfranc injury: how frequently does it get missed? And how can we improve? Injury 2007;38:856–60.

10. Gupta RT, Wadhwa RP, Learch TJ, et al. Lisfranc injury: imaging findings for this important but often-missed diagnosis. Curr Probl Diagn Radiol 2008;37:115–26.

11. Ly TV, Coetzee JC. Treatment of primarily ligamentous Lisfranc joint injuries: primary arthrodesis compared with open reduction and internal fixation. A prospective, randomized study. J Bone Joint Surg Am 2006;88:514–20.

12. Ramanujam CL, Zgonis T. Antibiotic-loaded cement beads for Charcot ankle osteomyelitis. Foot Ankle Spec 2010;3:274–7.

13. Capobianco CM, Stapleton JJ, Zgonis T. Soft tissue reconstruction pyramid in the diabetic foot. Foot Ankle Spec 2010;3:241–8.

14. Stapleton JJ, Zgonis T. Surgical reconstruction of the diabetic Charcot foot: internal, external or combined fixation? Clin Podiatr Med Surg 2012;29:425–33.

15. Zgonis T, Roukis TS, Polyzois VD. Lisfranc fracture-dislocations: current treatment and new surgical approaches. Clin Podiatr Med Surg 2006;23:303–22.

16. Wukich DK, Kline AJ. The management of ankle fractures in patient with diabetes. J Bone Joint Surg Am 2008;90:1570–8.

17. Wukich DK, Joseph A, Ryan M, et al. Outcomes of ankle fractures in patients with uncomplicated versus complicated diabetes. Foot Ankle Int 2011;32:120–30.

18. Jani MM, Ricci WM, Borrelli J Jr, et al. A protocol for treatment of unstable ankle fractures using transarticular fixation in patients with diabetes mellitus and loss of protective sensibility. Foot Ankle Int 2003;24:838–44.

19. Clement S, Braithwaite SS, Magee MF, et al. Management of diabetes and hyper-glycemia in Hospitals. Diabetes Care 2004;27:553–91.

Index

Note: Page numbers of article titles are in **boldface** type.

A

Abduction, provision for, 131
Abrasive wear, evaluation of, 129
Achilles tendon lengthening, for INBONE ankle replacement system failure, 233
Adhesive wear, evaluation of, 129
Agility ankle replacement system, **207–233**
    arthrodesis after, 220–222
    aseptic loosening of, 219
    cyst formation with, 210–211
    FDA-approved, 123
    fractures at, 219–220
    history of, 208–209
    osteolysis in, 152
    outcomes of, 135, 139, 209
    talar subsidence with, 211–216, 219
    tibial and talar subsidence with, 219
    tibial subsidence with, 216–219
American Orthopedic Foot and Ankle Surgeons Hindfoot-Ankle functional score, in cyst
    repair evaluation, **157–170**
Ankle Evolutive System, cyst formation in, repair of, **157–170**
Ankle replacement, revision of. See Revision total ankle replacement.
Anterior-posterior stability, 126
Anterolateral transfibular approach, to arthrodesis, 190
Antibiotics, for infection in INBONE ankle replacement system, 234
Arthrodesis
    for failed ankle replacement, **187–198**
        Agility system, 220–222
        challenges in, 188
        complications of, 204
        history of, 187–188
        INBONE system, 226–229
        outcomes of, 194–195
        postoperative care for, 193
        rehabilitation for, 193
        technique for, 189–193
    for osteolysis, 151–152
    outcomes of, 133
    tibiocalcaneal, for osteomyelitis and avascular necrosis, **251–256**
    tibio-talo-calcaneal, with intramedullary nail fixation, **199–206**
Arthrotomy, for INBONE ankle replacement system failure, 231–232
Aseptic loosening
    defects in, 149–150

Clin Podiatr Med Surg 30 (2013) 265–270
http://dx.doi.org/10.1016/S0891-8422(13)00014-1
0891-8422/13/$ – see front matter

Printed and bound by CPI Group (UK) Ltd, Croydon, CR0 4YY

03/10/2024

01040440-0016